"In Young's memoir, we are taken through the journey of deliverance from addiction and brought to the happy meeting of two soul-mates until tragedy strikes in the form of Alzheimer's at an unexpected, early age...The steadfastness and depth of the love of Mary Ann and Francis make this story ultimately an inspiring one."

MICHELLE DEMERS, POET AND EDUCATOR

"A heartfelt and heartbreaking memoir of love, loss, and indestructible devotion."

LAURIE ALBERTS, AUTHOR OF *Between Revolutions*

"Read this compelling and skillfully written memoir and be immediately captured by the honest writing and real life, unsettling story. Hold on tight until the end when you can finally exhale. Fuller Young bravely shares her humanness within the context of addiction, love and loss. A courageous, inspiring and authentic read that stays with you."

T. T. ZALINGER, MA, MSW

"In her wrenching new memoir, Plainly and Simply, Mary Ann Fuller Young zeroes in on the ravages of not one, but two insidious diseases: alcoholism and Alzheimer's...Despite the tragic nature of her subject matter, the ultimate tenor of the book is affirmative because of the resourcefulness and courage the author evinced confronting these illnesses."

DONALD ROWE,

PROFESSOR EMERITUS, CHAMPLAIN COLLEGE,

PRODUCER, DIRECTOR, ACTOR

PLAINLY & SIMPLY

A MEMOIR OF ALZHEIMER'S

Mary Ann Fuller Young

The beginning of love is to let those we love be perfectly themselves, and not to twist them to fit our image. Otherwise, we love only the reflection of ourselves we find in them.

THOMAS MERTON

The Champlain College Publishing Initiative provided support to the author in the creation of this book. The Champlain College Publishing Initiative has not undertaken any independent review or assessment of the quality, accuracy, completeness, currentness or other aspects of the content. Any views or opinions expressed in this book are the views or opinions of the author and do not necessarily represent those of the Champlain College Publishing Initiative, Champlain College, or its employees, trustees or representatives. The author alone is solely responsible for the content of the book and bears all responsibility for the publication of this book.

The names of people and some places have been changed for the sake of privacy.

Because of Francis

I am any woman, seventy-four years old. We could meet in the checkout lane at the supermarket. Comment about the pretty strawberries we are both buying. I am any woman, who saw my expectations about my future go awry. I am any woman, telling my story.

Table of Contents

Live and let live   9

Just a sip   13

First things first   19

Give time time   25

Interlude   33

Live in the now   35

Act as if   41

Now what?   49

Do the next best thing   63

A lesson   89

This too shall pass   95

One day at a time   111

Take it easy   115

Let go and let god   139

Turn it over   143

And so   157

Live and let live

My good buddy, as I had thought of Francis for years, invited me to go to the sea. To Spring Lake in particular, a quiet residential New Jersey shore town. Growing up in Connecticut, I had always gone to the beach; to the shore when I moved to New Jersey; to the ocean on trips to the Caribbean. But with this man, I would go to the sea. On an early summer day, nine years after I met Francis, the sun was rising and promising to shine all day. We left Allendale in Bup, his beige four-on-the-floor Honda—so named because of its license plate number, BUP 3671—and set out for a day at the sea.

We swam. Actually we bounced and bobbed about, as middle-agers are wont to do, when the chilling waves rolled in. Francis did the *New York Times* crossword puzzle. In ink. We ate long, skinny hot dogs with sauerkraut and gobs of spicy mustard and shared horrible green cotton candy. And we talked until we were hoarse.

Over time, similar day jaunts to the sea turned into overnight visits. Francis was eager to stay at a number of the charming, Victorian bed and breakfast establishments that we passed as we explored the towns along the Jersey shore.

Once, we stayed at the elegant old Spring Lake Inn. In the afternoon, we were bored with being at the pool and walked down the block to the sea. We strolled along the boardwalk, arm in arm, in step with each other, laughing, grinning. Every so often we stopped for a smooch and I peeked over Francis's shoulder to see if a passerby had slowed to watch. Later we sat in silence, close together on the scratchy, mustard-colored sand, and watched the waves dance a ballet as they tumbled into the shore.

Three, maybe four, years after we had started going to the sea, we stayed at Alice's Bed and Breakfast. In the middle of the night, I woke and sensed that Francis was gone. His clothes were neatly folded on the chair. His black leather Dopp kit was on the sink. I thought maybe he hadn't been able to sleep—an unusual thing for him—and he'd gone for a walk. No. Not without clothes. Why hadn't he woken me? I dressed and crept out of the B&B so as to not wake Alice or David, her policeman husband, and I held my breath as if that would help silence the noise of Bup's ignition. First, I searched for Francis in the blackness at the sea, and then I drove back and forth on the few streets that made up the eerie, lifeless, nighttime version of the town.

Back at the B&B, I tiptoed up the stairs to our empty room, praying all the while that Francis would be there. When he wasn't, I sat with my chin on the window ledge, stared into the creeping dawn, and listened for a telltale clue to interrupt the house sounds. At daybreak, I heard a snore. Down the hallway. We were the only guests on the second floor and all the bedroom doors were open. And I found Francis. Curled up, naked, in a room with twin beds. At breakfast with Alice and David, we decided Francis just turned the wrong way after he had gone to our bathroom, walked off down the hall, and found a bed. We blamed his loss of orientation and confusion on the antihistamine he had taken.

Of course, I wasn't willing to entertain any thoughts that would melt the magic we had found. I jumped at the easy explanation, but did I really buy the flimsy antihistamine excuse?

Francis and I explored many of the Jersey shore towns together. Cape May was the state's most famous resort spot and Francis wanted to take me there. He leafed through the bed-and-breakfast guidebook and chose the place for us to stay because he liked the large white wicker rockers on the wrap-around porch. While there, we rocked and rocked, but most of our time was spent on the sand at the sea. Francis had his puzzle to do and he pulled an easy, beginner puzzle book out of his L.L. Bean bag for me to try and told me to start by filling in the words I was sure of. I struggled. In pencil.

Riding home from Cape May in Bup, "By the Beautiful Sea" played on the radio. It was a keeper, written and composed by Ada Jones and Billy Watkins in 1914. "You and me, you and me, oh, how happy we'll be…I love to be beside your side, beside the sea, beside the seaside, by the beautiful sea!"

Just a sip

The end of an ordinary Sunday changed my life.

That morning, as usual, I poured my coffee and checked the Real Estate section in the Sunday edition of the local papers to confirm that my open house was advertised with a picture. As usual, I cut out the ad for the owners. My career in real estate had begun soon after my husband, Don, and I moved to New Jersey in 1976, in time for our son, Peter, to enter fifth grade.

That Sunday morning, after a breakfast of French toast, I drove to the A&P to purchase a frozen apple pie to bake at the open house. The home was an appealing Cape Cod, surrounded by mature oak trees. A cutting garden next to the cobblestone breezeway that led to the two car detached garage was in full bloom with irises, multi-colored gladiolas, yellow lilies, and ruby red dahlias. I gathered a sweet-smelling bouquet for the kitchen table.

The open house sign easily slid into the recently watered front yard. In preparation for visitors, I heated the oven for the pie—purchased primarily for its aroma—and turned on lights in all of the rooms, despite the ample natural light. The homeowners had taken my advice and had stashed away ordinary clutter. The furniture had recently been polished, leaving a touch of lemon oil in the air. Most homeowners expected their agents to hold numerous open houses, usually from 12:00 to 5:00 PM. on weekends. It was the most tedious part of my job, but the listings were lucrative. On this Sunday, I would rather have been playing golf or walking the dog.

It was quiet enough in the house to hear the buzz of the fish tank and I noticed when the elderly cat, Martin, climbed out of his bed to scratch in his litter box. An occasional car sped by. The sound of tires on the long and windy gravel driveway would serve to announce visitors so that I could graciously welcome them at the front door. The first three and a half hours were uneventful, tedious. My book didn't interest me; I was unable to concentrate on my crossword puzzle. I walked around the house, sat in an overstuffed armchair, moved to the antique brocade loveseat. My eyes were repeatedly drawn toward the drop-leaf coffee table holding the elegant Waterford crystal decanter, which was more than half full of a pale almond-colored liquid.

Just a sip. Why not just one little sip? I picked up one of the liqueur glasses, looked at the pattern, returned it to the silver tray, and started towards the kitchen in search of a soda. Then, I turned and went back to take a sip from the decanter. It was sweet. Warm. Another sip. I didn't know what I was sipping, only that it was sweet, warm, nice. A gulp. Other bottles were in the breakfront—open bottles of scotch, gin, and vodka. More sips. Sips of old favorites, depending on the period of my life and the season of the year, favorites before I had limited my drinking to vodka, believing it had no tell-tale odor.

Close to the time I was to put out the lights and get ready to leave, a man came and briefly looked through the house. We were standing in the kitchen with the slightly burned apple pie when he surprised me by offering to put the open house sign into the back of my Subaru. That had never happened before and I agreed to his kind offer. After he left, it occurred to me that he must have noticed I had been drinking and thought I needed some help. Would he report me to my boss? My muscles tightened.

Driving home would be a challenge, but my most nagging concern was how I would explain the now-empty glass decanter on the coffee table. The bottles in the breakfront, minus a sip here, a sip there, would escape detection. The cat. The cat knocked the decanter over. With his tail. Luckily, the decanter didn't break. I would call the homeowner and tell them that. Not today, as I would have ordinarily done after an open house to report about visitors and any prospective buyers. Tomorrow. I would call tomorrow.

I prided myself on being a highly professional and successful realtor. What the hell had happened to me? Surely I could have just one little sip. But one little sip was not enough. I needed more, had to have more, more sips, bigger sips.

Cautiously, I eased down the driveway to the road, a two-lane route, full of twists and turns that drivers took at high speed. I looked left and right, left again, right again, then held my breath as I pulled out of the driveway. Judging distances was impossible, despite squinting, closing one eye. There was no alternate, easy route back home. Good God, was I shaking? Too frightened to drive, I pulled over onto a gravel area and took a deep breath, relieved at finding a safe haven less than half a mile up the road. In a short time, maybe five minutes, a coupe pulled in behind me. Police? No. No lights. A car door slammed and a man appeared by my window. I twisted my head around and tried to determine if I knew him, but he was a stranger—pleasant-looking, middle-aged, wearing a dark suit with a busy flowered tie.

"Do you need help?" he asked.

"Yes," I said, "I need help."

The stranger suggested that he drive me home in my car and his wife would follow in their car. Greatly relieved, I agreed, gave directions, stared out the window.

"Have you ever heard anything about A.A.? Alcoholics Anonymous?" he asked.

"Some, yes. Some."

"You can get help there. There are meetings every day and evening all around this area. I think you should go and see about it. There is help for you."

"Thanks," I said. The important part of the stranger's message—that I could get help—slipped into my befuddled head.

The following morning, I recognized that I had completely lost control. I brushed my teeth and glanced into the mirror at a sad, sallow face, wrinkled beyond my forty-some years. What had happened? My friends described me as a vivacious, cheerful, athletic, caring woman; a tall, slender blond with clear blue eyes and a captivating smile, who played tennis, golf, sang, and danced with the vacuum cleaner. Where had she gone?

My daily drinking had begun soon after we lost our second son, baby boy Young, to hyaline membrane disease and other complications. I had seen our baby for only a moment, hadn't even held him before he was taken away to a critical care unit at Children's Hospital. My husband had gone along with our newborn and I had waited, alone, for reports on baby boy Young's slowly worsening condition. He died two and a half days later. At first, I did not feel it was my fault. But as time passed, I was haunted by thoughts that my previous drinking, smoking, and poor eating habits had caused baby boy Young's death.

After that, golf became a passion. I also turned my attention to fixing fancy gourmet dinners and frosty martinis. I have an indelible memory. In February 1968, I was standing in the living room of our railroad townhouse when it occurred to me that I did not have to wait for my husband to have a drink. I could drink alone.

In the early days of my solitary drinking in Virginia, I liked it. Hell, I loved it. Drunken Mary Ann and her booze; they danced and sang in the living room with Broadway show tunes blasting. I called friends, forgot I had called them, and called them back. Sure, I "managed" perfectly well.

Alcohol had an increasingly devastating and unpredictable effect on me as time drifted by. I was impervious to the progression and thought I was successful in my secret drinking. But what about my behavior? My flushed face? My red nose? Who was I kidding, trying to hide the proverbial elephant—more like a herd of them—in every room?

But I felt like I was in control. I had strict rules about my drinking. In the beginning it was not before 6:00 PM. That slid to 5:30 PM, then closer to 5:00. I would only drink at home. I was in control.

One fall day, knowing full well that I had to pick Peter up after soccer practice, I had a hefty slug, probably two, maybe more, around 4:00. I then drove the five miles or so to the school, early, before dark. I intended to sit and read in the car. It was difficult, then impossible to concentrate on my book. The vermouth's effect intensified quickly and the wait for Peter seemed interminable. When he finally arrived and as soon as I pulled out of the school parking lot, my anxiety level rose rapidly. We were almost home when, from the back seat, he said, "Mom, you've got to drive faster. You are creeping along." My rigid fingers gripped the steering wheel even tighter as I silently prayed. Dear God, please get us home, please. My heart rate escalated and I gritted my teeth. I was afraid of driving into the river that ran along the road or of hitting an oncoming car. I peered out the windshield, into black space. By the grace of God, we got home safely. Peter went right to the freezer, opening it to reveal my hidden coffee cup of vermouth. Before he went up to his room, he gave me a look I have never forgotten. I was not fooling him. We never discussed it further.

Why didn't I initiate a conversation with my son, make an apology? Who was this person I had become? Twenty-five years of drinking had claimed my self and knocked me low. I wanted to hide. Did

I try to quit drinking? No.

July 18, 1983—the day after my open house debacle, I attended an A.A. meeting. Barbara, whom I later learned was a long-time member of the A.A. fellowship and had helped many newcomers, noticed me and came over to say hello. In a laid-back and unassuming manner, she said she would be available if I needed her. "No, thank you, Barbara." Why would I need extra help? In time I learned to ask for help. In A.A. they say, "I can't, we can."

I was escorted to a meeting for beginners in a basement Sunday school room. What I heard that night was simple: "Don't drink. Go to meetings."

Bankers, lawyers, hookers, truck drivers, Mafia-trophy girlfriends, nuns, and judges attended the meetings. I asked everybody I met how to get sober, how to stay sober, and I got the same answers. "It's one day at a time. Don't drink. Go to meetings," they said. "It's a simple program for complicated people." I learned that it takes three to five days to get the alcohol out of my system and thus remove the physical need. The mental need was a different matter.

First things first

After a couple months of attending A.A. meetings in surrounding towns, I decided I would go to a beginners' meeting at the church in my hometown. Frank, a happy looking, well-dressed man, with a bounce to his step and a captivating smile, came over to welcome me during the coffee break. I had noticed him when I'd arrived and glanced around the room looking for an empty chair; he had a trench coat on his lap, rubbers on his shoes, and a well-worn, beige L.L. Bean shoulder bag at his feet. He told me he had been in A.A. for a year and a half, and was coffee maker at the Ramsey meeting on Friday nights. Coffee-making was a job his sponsor suggested he do for three months and he'd kept doing it. The following week, he saved me a seat at the meeting and after a month or so he said he could use some help in Ramsey, setting up the tables and fixing the coffee if I could, and wanted to, come early. That sounded good to me. Since it was important for me to get to a meeting every day, I traded my Friday morning meeting for the evening meeting.

Frank talked honestly, even about his embarrassing experiences, and I liked to listen to him. Sometimes, he told me, he went to two meetings a day. I understood that. Being in the company of alcoholics who were trying to achieve and maintain sobriety gave me confidence that I could succeed in improving my life. At the very least, meetings gave me confidence that I could stop drinking.

"Will you tell me your story?" Frank asked on the first night I went early to help set up for the Ramsey meeting.

"Sure, if you tell me yours," I answered.

We agreed to go for coffee and a bagel at the Waldwick Snak Shoppe after the Saturday meeting. I liked that he broke off a chunk of his plain, unsliced, untoasted bagel and offered it to me before he had a bite. We discussed growing up, alcohol in our families, drinking parties, college years, funny drinking stories, embarrassing drinking stories, kids, life.

Frank and I used different techniques to help us stay sober. He had always offered an alcoholic drink to guests at his house and he continued to do so. His mother had instilled that in him and his friends expected the gesture. Since joining A.A., he made sure he had a glass of Perrier with Rose's lime juice within easy reach. That was his crutch. It worked for him. Time and again, he referred to his drinking days as a past life, and he said repeatedly, "Drinking is not an option."

I started saying that same thing in my head.

My method to avoid drinking was different. "All the alcohol in my house is gone," I said. "Even the whole collection of liqueurs my in-laws gave us as Christmas presents. At first, I replaced bottles, but I quit that and when it was gone it was gone." My method was to guard against and avoid triggers. I focused on the catchword I had learned in the beginner meetings: HALT reminded me to avoid being hungry, angry, lonely, or tired. My day was revamped. I got home in the early afternoon and took a bath during what would have been my drinking time. I ate my favorite foods for dinner and went to meetings early. I sat outside and talked to whomever else came early to hang out in the safety zone that surrounded the meeting rooms. As my first year of A.A. passed, I developed a physical feeling of safety and relief when I arrived at a meeting.

In addition to my A.A. meetings, there were major changes at home. Peter left for college. Don took up training for the New York Marathon and went running many evenings, finishing long after I had gone to bed. Frequently, he went into the office during the weekend and I spent long hours involved with my real estate job.

To liven up our house and fill the void, we agreed to get a puppy, Churchill—an energetic, handsome yellow Labrador. And I adopted two kittens that had been living amid the potato bins and onion sacks outside the Ramsey farm store. The holiday periods, with Peter home from college and with visits from my mother-in-law, were pleasant, a welcome interlude to the lonely lifestyle Don and I had created.

In the rooms of A.A., numerous people commented that going to rehab or to detox had been the best thing that happened to them and that it gave them a jump start on living a life of sobriety. Some rehab programs were quite cushy, and very expensive. They typically lasted thirty days, but the length of stay was shortened as insurance companies cut back on their funding. Detox was usually for a week, in a hospital setting, and for some people it preceded going to rehab. Meds the patients received for the first three days made withdrawal from dependency on alcohol easier than having to white-knuckle it. To be honest, hearing these stories made me annoyed that Don had not taken any initiative to get medical help for me. I drank for a long time after it was pleasurable because it was too tough to fight my physical need.

We learned from each other's stories in A.A. I wanted to hear Frank's description about his detox days at Valley View hospital.

"Will you start at the beginning and tell me how you got to detox?" I asked Frank. "I'll buy you a bagel after the Saturday meeting."

"It's a date!"

Frank told me that after a neighborhood sing-along Christmas party he had slipped and fallen into a snow bank.

I interrupted: "Did your wife leave you there, in the snow?"

She had, he said. Then, in the morning, she had called Harv, a mutual friend and a longtime member of A.A., and they had driven Frank to Valley. He chuckled as he told me he had almost convinced the staff that he was there by mistake. Then he heard a number of other patients claiming the same thing after they had detoxed with meds and were feeling pretty good. It was there, in Ward 4, that Frank began to lose his terminal uniqueness, a type of denial that besets most alcoholics until they hear other people talk about feelings and experiences that they thought were unique to them. I began to see how that applied to me; lots of people had alcoholic families, felt abandoned and neglected in childhood, saw their self-worth diminish. Frank learned that some of the patients he originally referred to as lunatics, people back for the third or fourth time to detox, were, as he said, "just like me—drunks, having a rough time, trying to get sober. There went my terminal uniqueness!"

Before he left Ward 4, Frank made the decision that drinking was no longer an option for him. Period. He was sick and tired of being sick and tired. I understood. I was, too. Before he started A.A., he had a shot of vodka before he caught the train into Manhattan. He would drink his lunch, alone, ride home in the bar car, often miss his station stop, and would have to call his wife, Mattie, to come pick him up at the end of the train line in Suffern. After starting A.A., he avoided the bar car and took the bus home instead of the train.

Frank and I could laugh together and it felt good, but we knew our alcoholic antics were not funny at all. I became comfortable sharing stories that embarrassed me; Frank was nonjudgmental and so honest in discussing his own shortcomings that I learned I could tell him some of my history, my secret embarrassing episodes. His smile was reassuring. And he smiled so easily that I easily smiled back.

We didn't tell everything. I had much more to uncover. I had discovered how difficult it was to look into the past, to evaluate my behavior as well as the behavior of others. Getting sober was a significant step upward. But putting an end to my drinking was a surface solution. There was more to be done. It became clear to me that I placed a large chunk of blame for my situation, my "condition," outside of me—on heredity, on upbringing, on an assortment of excuses. This externalizing of blame had allowed me to rationalize my behavior. What if so-and-so had behaved differently? What if I had done X instead of Z? Did I repeatedly miss messages along the way by choosing to drink? Did I choose to forget and deny instead of paying attention?

During those first several months of going to A.A. meetings, I attended a real estate closing for a difficult transaction that I had been working on for months. The principals were assembled around a long table in the lawyer's office, and the secretary came in with champagne and a tray of glasses. It was a surprise. I was not prepared. Be polite, I thought. Just a sip.

"Yes, please," I told her. To fit in. To join the celebration. I had not yet learned how to say "No, thank you." It was easier to avoid situations where alcohol was being served.

Did I have seconds of champagne? How much did I have? I don't remember, but I do recall that driving towards my office to deliver my commission check, I got sidetracked by a ferocious need for alcohol. I was powerless. The nearest liquor store was a few miles down the road in HoHoKus, and I stood at the counter, balancing two bottles for an embarrassing stretch of time, trying to decide which bottle size to buy. Back behind the wheel, I drank from the bottle, securely hidden in a brown paper bag. By the time I was almost home, a mere four miles away, the bottle was empty. I drove to a different liquor store, but I don't remember anything after that. The A.A. slogan, "It's the first drink that gets you drunk," had confused me when I first heard it. After the champagne experience, I understood it completely. Two days later, I owned up to my slip at a meeting and was relieved to begin a new ninety meetings in ninety days.

I didn't have a drink for three weeks. Then I "forgot" there was never just a sip, never one single drink for me, and I arrived at a Sunday meeting tipsy, ready to explain to the group how A.A. could be better run. How arrogant I was. Fortunately, Frank detained me outside on the church steps and listened to me explain my theories until the break, at which time he went inside to find Barbara to help deal with me. She was the picture of calm, with her short, dark brown hair, sturdy build, and deeply pitched, ready laugh. She convinced me to go home, and she followed me there and walked me to the door. It was time to take her up on her offer of help. I asked her to be my sponsor.

With her encouragement—we talked on the phone frequently—I continued to go to meetings and read the A.A. literature. I repeated the serenity prayer often: "God, grant me the serenity to accept the things I cannot change, courage to change the things I can, and wisdom to know the difference."

Give time, time

Fourteen months after my first A.A. meeting, I got my ninety-day pin. I knew that I still had to work hard to maintain my life-saving journey to a sober life. It took me some time to understand, and even cherish, the numerous slogans used in A.A., slogans that I had thought were so hokey at first. "I can't, we can." "One day at a time." "Live and let live." "Let go and let God." "Easy does it." "There are no coincidences in A.A." "Give time, time." And the granddaddy of them all: "Don't drink. Go to meetings."

Fascinating people, with extraordinary stories to tell, landed in the rooms of A.A., and the people I met there had a lot to do with my staying and striving for sobriety. Clark, an ace fighter pilot who still wore his boots and an old leather jacket, became a close friend. He was older, probably in his sixties, and ran the Saturday A.A. meeting at the rehab clinic in Ridgewood. "We all need to give some payback to this program, you know," he said, and invited me to come to the meeting and tell my story. He strongly encouraged me to be a speaker. I was what was referred to as a high-bottom drunk; I still had family, a home, food on the table, a job; I had not committed a grievous crime while under the influence of alcohol. There are many levels of drunks, but a drunk is a drunk. Once I got past my initial nervousness, it was easy to stand in front of an A.A. group and talk. I latched onto the concept that alcoholism was a disease. I spoke about my experiences with trying to have just a sip and my slip at the real estate closing, which taught me the value of the slogan, "It's the first drink that gets you drunk." Some people nodded their heads in agreement when I described how horrible it felt to have no power over my own behavior.

Barbara, my sponsor, frequently asked me to join a group of A.A. members that went to Howard Johnson's after the Ramsey Friday night meeting. I usually pleaded tiredness, explaining that my job in real estate sales was very time consuming, but on my forty-seventh birthday, almost three years after I had first walked into the rooms of A.A, I agreed to go. When I looked up from the menu, having decided on black coffee and a single scoop of unadorned peach frozen yogurt, Frank—chunky, solid, smiling Frank—had joined our group and was unabashedly ordering a banana split. He beamed at his scoops of chocolate, coffee, and Buttercrunch ice cream, covered with whipped cream, topped with three red cherries, snuggled in between a split banana, afloat in a sea of fudge sauce. He offered me the first bite, winked, and said, "Come to the Promises meeting in Manhattan and I'll take you to Schrafft's for a banana split." There are twelve promises in the big book of A.A. Each promise describes what can happen as a result of leading a sober life. It was not the first time Frank suggested I go to that meeting. It was the first time he offered the ice cream. Barbara overheard Frank's invitation and said I should go, that a Promises meeting would add an important dimension to my sobriety.

The next morning, after the Waldwick speakers meeting, Frank and I were sitting on the stone wall, enjoying the sunshine and the vibrant fall foliage. I liked to look at him. He was distinguished-looking, had a tiny scent of spice. A solid sort of guy with broad shoulders, he had played fullback on his high school football team, and had played ice hockey in college until he discovered he preferred the drinking club. That shot his hockey game. He was always immaculately groomed. He used handkerchiefs and always had a small silk scarf in his breast pocket. He was balding and graying at the temples. His eyes, a deep powder blue, smiled. He cared about others and did hospice work. Frank held doors for strangers, and would tip his hat if he was wearing one. What I liked best, though, was when he looked at me; I sensed that he cared deeply, about my thoughts, my concerns, me. Simply said, the attention he paid me made me feel important. I basked in it.

I knew other men named Frank, but this man was different and I asked him if I could call him by his given name: Francis. "Sure, hon." It made me feel like we had an exclusive link.

"Who's your best friend?" I spontaneously asked, as we sat on the sun-warmed wall.

"My wife," he said.

"I envy you," I blurted out.

In a flash, I realized that I wished my husband was my best friend. Suddenly, I saw that as I had racked up three-and-a-half sober years, Don and I still continued to pass, staying on our individual paths.

Francis's answer surprised me. Maybe I expected him to say his sponsor, Harv, was his best friend. Maybe I wanted him to say I was his best friend. I realized I was jealous. At any rate, I felt that he had defined our relationship with that answer: we were very good friends, helping each other stay sober.

"How about I come to the Promises meeting, finally, after the holidays? See what it's all about," I said.

"I'll meet you there any time you can come." He smiled the kind of smile that flickered in his eyes.

On a rainy, gray January morning, I drove to the train station to go to Manhattan and the Promises meeting. Worried about missing the train, I left home twenty minutes early to allow for my general state of agitation, parking, and visiting the ladies room. As a teen growing up in Fairfield, Connecticut, I had often gone into the city for shopping on Fifth Avenue or for a matinee so I had some familiarity with Grand Central Station. Still, it was new for me to be traveling alone, on an adventure. It was exciting.

I bought a local newspaper, chose a window seat, watched commuters board and disembark at the many stops along the way, and peered out the grimy windows into suburban backyards with naked trees, dried up leaves, and scattered toys from warmer play days. There was something about the train ride, being alone, away from home and my usual environment that made it safe to peek at my life, to explore where I had been, and speculate about where I might be going. During the ride, I realized that it took a large amount of my energy to pretend—to the world and to myself—that my marriage was a good one. Clearly, Peter had become the glue in our family of three.

Grand Central Station was big, beautiful, and bustling with the energy and excitement I associated with New York City. It was invigorating just to join the crowd. As I hustled down the street, Francis was standing by the side door to the First Presbyterian Church on 68th Street, waving to me, smiling. I was very happy to see him.

A group had assembled in the reception area, waiting for the small elevator, a cranky-looking old thing with a black metal safety door. Aside from Francis's, there were no familiar faces. The elevator clunked and bounced as it settled into its first floor niche. We clambered in, turned to face the front, adopted the standard elevator gaze. At each floor the elevator slowed, laboring with its heavy load, then got a little burst of energy to lift upwards and continue to the fifth floor. We filed out of the elevator, politely, two by two. Lots of people—young people, even some teens, oldsters, banker types, office girls, CEOs, blue-collar workers—in a huge hall, greeted each other and got themselves settled on the grey metal folding chairs that were lined up in semi-circular rows, not unlike a revival meeting. The homeless, with their ripped and dirty canvas backpacks and bedrolls, sat on the floor and leaned against the twelve-foot pine paneled walls. In the front of the room, there were three large posters with the Twelve Promises of Alcoholics Anonymous:

1   If we are painstaking about this phase of our development, we will be amazed before we are half way through.

2   We are going to know a new freedom and a new happiness.

3   We will not regret the past nor wish to shut the door on it.

4   We will comprehend the word serenity and we will know peace.

5   No matter how far down the scale we have gone, we will see how our experience can benefit others.

6   That feeling of uselessness and self-pity will disappear.

7   We will lose interest in selfish things and gain interest in our fellows.

8   Self-seeking will slip away.

9   Our whole attitude and outlook on life will change.

10   Fear of people and economic insecurity will leave us.

11   We will intuitively know how to handle

situations that used to baffle us.

12   We will suddenly realize that God is
      doing for us what we could not do for
      ourselves.

Are these extravagant promises? We think not. They are being fulfilled among us, sometimes quickly, sometimes slowly. They will materialize if we work for them.

Two dynamic speakers, Greg and Elaine, with very different backgrounds and histories, told how the promises had infiltrated their lives. Greg, a handsome, well-dressed CEO, related how difficult it had been for him to remember how to do things that were essential to his job. A friend confronted him and told him he was on the brink of being fired if he didn't stop the noontime boozing. Elaine, the other speaker, smiled and showed off the new teeth that she had finally managed to get after she moved out of her battered cardboard box on the street and got a job at a Reed's Drug Store. When she thanked everyone in the room for standing by her for the twelve years she had been coming to this meeting, she became teary.

In spite of being at a different type of meeting, in a new location and city, it made me feel that I was in the right place, and that I would like to come back. The meeting ended in the customary way. Everyone stood in a huge circle, joined hands, and recited the promises before adding, "Keep coming back. It works if you work it, so work it."

What had taken me so long? It was just an A.A. meeting, wasn't it? I was thinking about returning the following week and almost missed hearing Francis say "I have reservations at the Rock Plaza for lunch, if that would please you. We could watch the skaters."

"Yes, Francis, thanks." Lunch had never crossed my mind and I was flattered by the unexpected invitation to the upscale Rockefeller Plaza restaurant.

Within a few steps, we were at the curb of Sixty-Eighth Street. Francis took my hand. Firmly. He didn't let go. I noticed and wondered about it, but for less than a split second. This was different, confusing, more than just meeting up to go to an A.A. meeting. I was getting a mixed message from my "best buddy."

The Rock Plaza was a charming place for lunch. The waiter called Francis by name. That impressed me. By the time our entrée arrived, I was comfortable being with him in this new and different setting, away from the rooms of A.A. I wondered what he thought of being at the Rock Plaza with me, but I didn't ask. It was important to me to make a good impression on this special man, a man who was making me feel like a special lady.

The conversation at lunch centered, excitedly, about starting a Promises meeting in our area in New Jersey. It seemed like we could work well together as a team. Yes, together.

There didn't need to be a street to cross for Francis to quickly take my hand as we headed to Schraft's. We were about the same height and easily fell in step, keeping pace with each other. Don always walked off way in front of me and I had to frequently call to him to wait for me.

At Schrafft's, a New York City institution, the waitress brought two cups of coffee, and one very large banana split, with clouds of whipped cream spilling over the sides of the dish, two long handled silver spoons, extra fudge sauce. Francis held out the first bite for me. It was delectable.

Interlude

Peter and his longtime girlfriend, Amy, joined Don and me at our Jeffersonville, Vermont vacation house for a June weekend. Don and I had purchased the lot when Peter was at college, mainly because of the unobstructed view of Mount Mansfield, the highest of Vermont's Green Mountains. We had since built the large, three-bedroom Yankee barn, with a Jacuzzi and a sauna for skiers who rented the place for much of the winter. The house sat on a hilltop surrounded by five acres at the end of an unpaved country road. The natural setting, with copses of white birches—my favorite—was gorgeous any time of year.

I was sitting on the deck in the June sun, Don was pruning a tree, and Amy was quietly perched on the deck railing. Peter joined us. They both talked at the same time to explain they had chosen July 6 as a wedding day and—surprise!—wanted the venue to be in New Jersey.

"Is that okay, Mom?" they asked. I was overjoyed, and loved the challenge of the short amount of time to pull everything together. "Sure, that's okay! It's great!" I said.

We buckled down to make it happen. Francis had been part of his daughters' weddings in the past couple of years and we often talked about how it felt to have a child enter this new phase of life. We had mixed emotions about the milestone.

I loved doing the wedding preparations, but the best part was having Peter and Amy around. It was the first—and last—time I made a huge number of tiny meatballs, which I served at the rehearsal dinner held in our backyard. Don borrowed an ice cream vending cart for serving beer and wine and rigged up speakers for music. We danced happily on our driveway.

Live in the now

During the next three years, my friendship with Francis deepened as we chatted before and after meetings. We were of the same vintage and had been in marriages for thirty-two or -three years with, as is said, a good deal of water over the dam. Aside from never-ending discussions about A.A., we talked about what was going on in our families over bagels at the Snak Shop in Waldwick, baked potatoes at Wendy's in Ramsey, and frozen yogurt at TCBY in Glen Rock. The short of it was that Francis was a proud papa and beamed when he spoke about his daughters, Claudia and Carolyn, and his son, Ronald, and their antics and accomplishments. Ronald had landed a well-paying job and worked in both Manhattan and California. Claudia had married her hometown sweetheart and moved to Alexandria, Virginia. Carolyn was engaged and wedding plans were underway. I talked about Peter graduating from college and law school and moving on to a position in a Boston law firm. We compared notes on how it felt to have a child leave home and begin an independent life.

We frequently met for lunch in New York City, with or without an A.A. meeting in New York City. It was wonderful to have a reason to dress up, buy some new clothes, get my hair done. I was paying attention to what I ate, feeling healthy, and looking better than I had for years. It was easy to laugh again, to smile. We walked on Fifth Avenue and went to museums. In no time at all, it began to feel perfectly natural to be together doing these things. As an executive search recruiter, Francis could have business lunches with anyone, could entertain clients anywhere, and he frequently traveled out of town for his job. He was his own boss, working on commission, as was I in real estate. I fashioned a professional and comfortable client persona for myself when we were together in public places in Manhattan and where Francis was recognized.

A couple years after our first lunch date and my first Promises meeting, Francis invited me into Manhattan for lunch at P.J. Clark's. He had been avoiding his old haunts and his associated memories of drinking his lunch alone, and now wanted to revisit a few of those places. Sober. With me. I watched an aristocratic-looking elderly man, dressed to the nines and using a cane with a polished silver handle, cautiously sit down at the table next to us at P.J.'s. The waiter greeted him and asked, "The usual?" The gentleman nodded and fidgeted. His double martini arrived. He left it on the table. It made me uncomfortable to see him bend over to drink it through a straw, which the waiter had known to bring. Soon, the gentleman was ready for the second double martini. He could manage to pick that one up. It was hard not to stare. And it was easy to think, "There, but for the grace of God, go I."

That same winter, out for lunch at the King Cole Bar, we chose the crab croquette special. Most of the other patrons were business-men, indulging in the other daily special: two signature cocktails for the price of one. Francis paid the bill, like he always did, with one of the ten or more credit cards he carried deep in his left pants pocket. While paying he added, "You know, the card companies don't care if you just pay a very small amount each month."

Of course, later, I thought Francis's comment was odd. Had he just become aware of this common credit card company policy? He didn't seem to be joking! When I was a teenager my father instructed me in financial matters and taught me the perils of accruing late charges and interest on interest. It had been instilled in me that debts needed to be paid promptly and never should I take on a debt I did not expect to be able to pay. Didn't Francis pay his bills in full each month like I did? The possibility that he was considering paying just a "small amount" on his credit cards seemed inconceivable to me, but I didn't probe. I liked this man and didn't want to appear nosy or disapproving. Besides, I thought Francis gave the impression that he was in a comfortable financial position.

Francis's credit cards were wrapped in wads of pink memo slips and secured with an elastic band.

"What are all those pink slips?" I asked.

"Oh, memos that remind me who called, what they said and what I said." Francis spent much of his time away from his desk and worked from home and on the road. Maybe, I thought, that was why he lugged his L.L. Bean bag everywhere; it must be full of files. His portable office.

I turned up the collar on my mink coat in anticipation of the chilling winter wind, and we wove between the crowded tables towards the elevator. As we approached the lobby, I sensed that Francis's arm was raised. He followed me closer than usual. Too close. Had I turned around, we would have collided. It crossed my mind that I could escape the slightly uncomfortable situation and go to the ladies' room, but I had just been there.

In the lower level elevator arcade, we were alone. I tapped the elevator button on the brocade floral wallpaper and the door slid back. In unison, we moved into the cherry-walled cocoon. A burned out bulb in the gaudy chandelier caught my eye, and as I glanced up, Francis kissed me. I was surprised. But I discovered I was a very willing participant. Bells rang from impatient patrons on the upper floors of the Saint Regis Hotel, but Francis had silently locked the elevator in a stationary position. Although there had been fleeting pecks on the cheek, at holiday times during the past years, this was our first real kiss. It didn't matter that we were in our mid-fifties. A first kiss is a first kiss.

One kiss led to another. My attitude was to try to simply enjoy the adventure while it happened, one day at a time, to take it easy and not complicate it by trying to map out any future. I was practicing the principles of A.A., paying attention to the slogans. "Let go, let God."

One evening, at the famous Stage Deli in Manhattan, we indulged in gigantic bacon, lettuce, and tomato sandwiches and cheesecake to starve for. The only time Francis ever made a comment about the price of anything was there. "Pretty pricey," he said. And it was.

Out of the blue, Francis acted peculiar when he met me at the bus station in Times Square for a late-February lunch date. He didn't chatter amicably and act like he was happy to see me. Rather, he hardly said a word and his customary smile was replaced with a look of pre-occupation. I made small talk but he was mostly unresponsive. When we arrived at our favorite restaurant, Café des Artistes on West Sixty-Seventh Street, Francis was uncharacteristically annoyed that our usual table, number twenty-one, in a private alcove, was unavailable. It was fine with me if we sat elsewhere, but not for Francis. He chose for us to wait at the bar. We nursed our Perriers with lime. Silence sat between us. As we were finishing our rare poached salmon Francis peered over his horn-rimmed glasses, focused into the distance, and spoke hesitantly: "I don't know how to tell you. But A.A. is a program of honesty and...."

My insides collapsed. My face slid into pale, the corners of my lips turned downward. I held my breath. I feared Francis was moving away, taking a job somewhere else, was ill, or I didn't know what. What if we could no longer see each other? A dagger popped into my gut as my perpetual concerns over being abandoned were kindled. To top it all off, I glimpsed a man in a tan raincoat sprinting across the street, flashing his nude private parts. Despite the distraction, I heard this:

"Plainly and simply, I have to tell you I am in love with you. Plainly and simply. I have been trying to tell you that for a long time."

My composure was shot to hell. I responded, "Oh, that's okay."

Or at least that's what Francis later told me I said. Our taxi inched along on Fifth Avenue. Francis pulled me close, kissed me with a wandering tongue.

My dreamy eyes were closed, then they popped open. I pushed Francis's black cashmere scarf off my nose and asked, "Can you support me in the way I am accustomed to...?"

My question trailed away when he indicated yes and we returned to the big kiss.

Later, I also asked, "If it weren't for me, would you be working on your marriage?"

Francis's answer was emphatic: "No, I've been working on my marriage for thirty-three or more years. Long enough. A past life."

He got out of the cab to go back to his office for what was left of the afternoon and said, "I want you to be part of my dream for a new beginning. I'll tell you all about it." He pushed a ten-dollar bill into my leather-gloved hand to more than pay for my short ride to the Port Authority where I would catch the bus home.

"See you tomorrow," he mouthed as he put his hand to his chin and blew me air kisses.

"Whoowee," exclaimed the burly taxi driver. "That sure ain't no hubby."

"He's my boyfriend. Yep, my boyfriend." Plainly. Simply.

Horns blasted. The driver cussed in an unrecognizable language, extended his middle finger out the window and jerked into the perpetual New York City traffic.

The next morning, as I was drinking my coffee, the lyrics "It's wonderful, it's marvelous, that you should care for me" kept repeating in my head. More than anything I wanted to talk to Francis, but it was only a little after five o'clock AM. and he, most likely, was on the bus heading into his office. I was smitten and ready to take the leap and be in giddy love, for today, for one day at a time. I couldn't wait to tell Francis that, but I did wait, I waited until I saw him again a few days later. In front of the City Center, I hopped out of a cab, jumped over the puddles forming from the teeming rain, and ran into Francis's arms. "I love you! I love you!" Francis clutched me, held me tight as if we were one, and beamed about my happiness, our happiness.

Act as if

Don and I were going to New Hampshire for the weekend for a family wedding. I was in my study, getting things in order. I was feeling quite nervous about telling Don my plans to drive up early Friday morning, alone, and stay at our vacation house for a few days after the weekend of family festivities. While I was at the wedding, Francis would be at Tupper Lake for a family vacation. We expected to get together.

I frowned, and from my study called out my travel intentions to Don while he was shaving.

He heard me.

"No. No, Mary Ann. We are not taking separate cars. We are driving together this afternoon when I get home from work. Come here. We have to talk."

It was ordinary behavior for Don to tell me what to do and it was ordinary behavior for me to do it. I sat at the foot of the huge unmade bed. It had been Don's idea to put two double beds together. I heard the water splashing in the sink and Don saying that he knew about Frank.

At first, I wondered what he knew, and then I wondered how he found out. But I couldn't really ask him that, could I? What could I do? I knew. I could shut up. That's what I could do. Just shut up and listen.

As I recall Don added that he assumed it was a joke, offered forgiveness, and said that I had to give up Frank.

In almost a whisper, with barely any forethought, I said, "No. No, I am not giving up Frank." I shut up then. I did not add that I was not the least bit interested in Don's brand of forgiveness. Nor did I believe he could forgive.

Of course, years later I understood that this was a pivotal moment for me, a moment that essentially ended my marriage.

I took deep breaths around the rocks in my stomach. As soon as Don left for the office, I called Francis and told him what happened. We agreed to meet at the Sagamore Inn at Lake George on the Monday afternoon after the wedding. The A.A. slogan, "Fake it until you make it," dictated my behavior that weekend: I buried my inner turmoil as best I could and worked to appear calm. I acted as if everything was fine. I said the serenity prayer in my head more times than I could ever count. The wedding reception was in the bride's garden. When the disk jockey played "I Just Called to Say I Love You" or "Lady In Red," songs that Francis and I shared, I scooted off to the ladies' room or to the swing by the trellis of pink roses to be alone. It was uncomfortable when guests asked when Don and I were going to dance, and I imagined being in his arms, playing the happy couple charade.

Finally, it was Monday. Francis, wearing white ducks, a pale blue polo shirt, his canvas hat crammed in his back pocket, met me in the parking lot of the exquisite Sagamore Inn. His hand found mine and we walked along the stone path through the multitude of gardens with their pink, red, yellow blooms to a concrete bench over-looking Lake George. We sat. I cried the whole afternoon.

"I'll figure this out," Francis said. "Can you meet me back here on Wednesday?"

A welcome calm settled over me as I returned to Jeffersonville to wait for Wednesday.

Francis was standing in the parking lot, sporting his signature grin, happy to see me. Before we even got to the door of the Saga-more Inn he said, "We'll get married! If you'll have me!"

Of course, this was the first time Francis mentioned marriage. We would both need divorces. I knew that I wanted to be with him, but I didn't want to scare him away. It didn't feel right for me to introduce marriage. After all, the way I learned was boy asks girl, right?

My answer was yes.

There was no room in my head or my heart to even think about what complications might occur.

We went into the coffee shop and ordered a turkey club, no mayo for him and a BLT on rye with extra lettuce for me. Francis got up and came to my side, went down on one knee, put his hand on his back for support, and said, "I love you, plainly and simply, Mary Ann. Marry me, marry me."

Patrons clapped and cheered. My whole being clapped and cheered.

It was August 18th, 1993.

The next day, Francis returned to his family at Tupper Lake for the remainder of their vacation week and I went to the vacation house. At the end of the week, it was time to return to New Jersey, and to go to Diane's wedding on Sunday. With Francis. I had be-come Diane's sponsor in A.A. Her daughter was in rehab and it had been agreed that she could leave and attend her mother's wedding if she had a chaperone. Francis and I were to pick her up at rehab, keep an eye on her, and drive her back at the end of the reception.

The morning of that Sunday, I got an "all hell has broken loose" phone call from Francis. He had to stay home in the morning and would not be able to go to the A.A. meeting with me as planned, but he would meet me at one o'clock PM. to go to the wedding. Mattie had been looking for a Snickers bar in his L.L. Bean bag and had come across a card I had given Francis that said, "I love you, in the morning, in the night, etc., but best of all I love you naked." Needless to say, she wanted some explanations and was calling the children to arrange for discussions with Francis on the phone.

Dressed and ready to go out the door a little before one o'clock PM, I stopped to answer the ringing phone.

"I don't know why I am calling you," Mattie said.

"I don't know why either," I said.

Diane was a beautiful bride and her daughter behaved appropriately. Francis and I danced under a black balloon of tension, wondering what would erupt next. Don knew I was going to the wedding—an A.A. related event—but he hadn't known I was going with Francis.

Of course, I planned to get a divorce, but I was not so sure that Francis would be able to follow through and get his. Thirty-three years of marriage, through thick and thin and three children, had weight. An Ann Lander's column that claimed men rarely left their long-term marriages stuck in my mind.

Francis and I visited a well-respected divorce lawyer together. "Strike while the iron is hot," as the saying goes. It was September 7th, 1993. The lawyer required a three thousand dollar retainer fee for both of us. I paid.

Months of fretful, upsetting discussions with his wife and his adult children occurred at Francis's house during this period. I was not privy to any details. Finally, it was agreed that Mattie, rather than Francis, would file for the divorce.

When Don told me to give up Francis and I had said no, I asked Don to move out of our marital home. He refused. I moved into the guest room. We existed like strangers, rarely seeing each other. As soon as the tenants vacated one side of the little antique, ivy-covered stone duplex in Ho-Ho-Kus that a partner and I had purchased as an investment property, I would move there. Don was visiting his mother when I called to tell him I was leaving. It was December 29th, 1993.

The day the movers loaded and carted away the small amount of my furniture that would fit in the Ho-Ho-Kus house, Don sat on the front steps and watched. It was awful. Upsetting. Frightening. A mammoth boulder lodged in my lungs.

The following year and a half was full of turmoil for Francis. And it was unsettling for me. He only talked about fragments of his difficulties at home with Mattie and his children, but, too frequently, he sat at my kitchen table with a tepid cup of coffee and cried. Repeatedly, he professed that we would, one day, be together. We had agreed that we did not need to wait for divorces to be finalized to begin living together. The day arrived eighteen months after I had moved into Ho-Ho-Kus. He knocked on the red door.

"Hello!" he beamed. "I'm here to be with you, forever and ever, if you will have me! I'm yours!"

He was carrying white and blue button-down shirts on hangers and a brown leather Dopp kit.

As much as I wanted to believe in us being together in a permanent arrangement, I had my doubts. I felt better when he brought over his suits, ties, ratty old moccasins, and summer clothes from his garage, where Mattie had put them, and managed to neatly arrange them in the miniscule closet in my office. Both of our divorces were in progress.

Within a short time after Francis moved in, things gradually changed. Francis gradually changed. He still phoned me frequently from the office as he had been doing for many years just to say hello, just to say I love you, but often also to ask if we had plans for the evening or if I wanted him to pick up something from the market. Occasionally, he would call again, as if he had forgotten we had spoken earlier. It was nice, though, to hear his voice any time of day.

Of course, at the time I didn't try to describe it or understand it beyond noting a difference in his behavior. Putting words to it, I would have to say Francis seemed a little preoccupied. Not all the time, but sometimes.

Our living arrangement was easy. We had no need for further courtship; we fit together and we knew it. Francis wasn't much good at the stove, but he would fix a decent cup of coffee, or go out to buy bagels, and he was masterful with the vacuum cleaner and especially the broom. He emptied waste baskets without being asked. The dozen or so red, mauve, and pink geranium plants that he purchased and placed on the stone steps by the front door thrived under his loving touch and produced gorgeous blooms as if they were competing to see which plant could be bushier and prettier.

Together, we made a trip to the farm store in Ramsey, where kittens were usually available to go to a home. We chose Sagamore and Philadelphia to liven up our little abode. Months later, we added the most gorgeous Labrador retriever puppy, Barnes, so named because we picked him out from the kennel—or rather he picked me out—after we had been to the Barnes Foundation art exhibit in Philadelphia.

Shortly after Francis had moved in with me in Ho-Ho-Kus, he received the news that his daughter Claudia and her husband, Tilden, were expecting a long-awaited baby. Francis lit up and bubbled with enthusiasm about being a grandpa. We shopped together and picked out a baby's first year book. When the gift was returned, unopened, with a note in big, black, bold letters on the package from Tilden—Do not contact us ever again—Francis was distraught and I was angry. Francis made a number of phone calls to Claudia that went unreturned. Sadly, attempts to visit the grandbaby did not materialize.

Francis commuted to work in Manhattan and often casually commented on his unsuccessful attempts to meet his son, Ronald, for lunch. I sensed that it bothered Francis not to be in close touch with his children. Ronald did come to visit, once, with his girlfriend, Lisa. He was a tall and handsome young man with dark hair. The occasion was uncomfortable for me. Ronald was standoffish and I felt he had come to check out the situation, to see what his father was up to. We went out for dinner at the Spanish restaurant in Allendale. Despite having lived in Spain and favoring the cuisine, Francis barely ate a morsel or spoke a word.

Now what?

Everything about the move added up to being a screaming nightmare. On the day of departure, the movers phoned and woke us at 7:00 AM to say they would arrive early, within a half hour. By the time the huge Mayflower truck rumbled in, brushing the graceful old elms that canopied Lakewood Avenue, and eased up in front of the home where we had lived for the past year and a half, dark clouds had gathered. The movers carted things to the truck at breakneck speed. Francis left to get gas and pick up his shirts at the cleaners, an errand I thought he should have done sooner, but I didn't say so.

"Don't forget my sweater," I yelled as he drove off.

He returned bearing $7 worth of toilet paper, a bargain a stranger at the gas station had pointed out to him. Good God, how would we cram this in our overflowing cars? Which mover's question needed to be answered first? Would we ever get the hell out of here?

Francis waited for my attention. From behind his back, he produced a red rose. "For my beautiful lady," he beamed.

"Is it too late at my age to make a dream come true?" Francis said one day. "I'd like to open my own executive search firm. It doesn't take rocket science to do it, hon. You can be my assistant." He had mentioned this dream of his before, but now he was ready to act.

"Yes. Yes. Do it, Francis. Fifty-six is young; we are young, we can do it." I believed in my Francis. Truth be told, I had fallen madly in love with this man. His dream could be my dream.

Francis had left the corporate world and been successful in the executive search field for fifteen years in New York City. In 1994, *Money Magazine* identified the Research Triangle, an area between Durham and Raleigh, North Carolina that was rapidly expanding with corporate headquarters as the number one place to live and work. That location would be perfect for an executive search firm, and it was where Francis wanted to go. He put out feelers and quickly got an offer from a New Jersey firm to head up a satellite office in the Research Triangle Park. This was a reasonable stepping-stone to setting up his own company and would provide Francis with an opportunity to learn the lay of the land. And he would be salaried.

We traveled to Raleigh-Durham to explore the possibilities. The more we saw of North Carolina, the more we liked it. During our search for a reasonable office space, Francis would step aside and let me ask most of the questions. Though a little surprising, it was reasonable considering my experience in real estate. We visited a variety of neighborhoods, inspecting potential rental houses from the outside and found a charming two-story on a cul-de-sac near a little lake with ducks. It was in Carrboro, at the fringe of the university town of Chapel Hill. It would be available for us in June. Perfect. That day, the sun was shining. The sky was an incredible Easter-egg blue. A Carolina blue.

But the penny didn't fall in the slot.

The New Jersey firm that had offered Francis the satellite position in North Carolina suddenly changed its plans about being involved. Francis didn't seem overly concerned, which bothered me. And he didn't have a ready explanation. For whatever reason, I didn't press him.

A memory of an evening when we were in New York City, near the office where Francis had worked for over ten years, came to mind. On the way to Avery Fisher Hall in Lincoln Center, Francis stopped at a corner, stood still, and mumbled, "I'm confused. I don't know which way to go." I read the street signs to him. He acted as if he had never heard of Columbus Avenue. Though it seemed strange to me, my thoughts were diverted as he quickly pulled me close for a giant bear hug and said, "Oh, well. This is being in love!" Perhaps during a meeting with the New Jersey firm Francis had had a similar lapse of memory or went off on a tangent and they decided not to hire him for the proposed satellite project.

"Now what, my love? Do we still go to North Carolina? Do it on our own?" he asked.

"I'll pack," I said.

I was very concerned about our animals amidst the commotion with the packers and movers going in and out of the house. Barnes was safely secured, tied to a tree where he could watch. The neighbors graciously agreed to keep our skittish kittens in their guest room until we were ready to leave because I was betting we would not be able to locate them when we needed to. The details of why Francis let the kittens out of the neighbors' house when he returned from the gas station eluded me. Now, as expected, we had a big problem. Sagamore ran off to hide in some hole and refused to come near us until he got hungry enough and the slimy, ripe bologna I was tempting him with smelled too good to ignore. He clawed my leg, badly, bloodily, when I finally grabbed him and got him into his carrier case. We drove to the emergency room. I needed twelve stitches and a tetanus shot. Francis held my hand.

Relief engulfed me as I tuned in classical music and settled myself behind the wheel of my Volvo filled with suitcases, Barnes, and the kittens, my vocal company for the ten hour drive to North Carolina. I kept looking in my rearview mirror to make sure Francis was following in his car, which was crammed with gear and his shirts on hangers, like a traveling salesman.

Of course, it happened bit by bit that I started watching out for Francis and checking to see if he needed any help. That's what you do when you love someone. Take care of him.

Our first stopping point was for a late lunch at the Betsy Ross Rest Area. At the check out cash register, Francis fumbled with his pockets. I giggled, nervously, and had to ask him if he were planning on buying my lunch as he always did, always had. The situation felt weird, confusing. "Sure, sure," he mumbled and put back a Coke that was on his tray. As we ate, we reviewed the directions to our motel in Maryland in case we got separated en route.

"See you there," I said, with fake cheerfulness, and started my car. But Francis hung around by the door, smiled a lot, paused, and finally asked, "Can you loan me some money for the tolls? I am flat out. Just keep a tally, hon, and I'll pay you back. Everything I have is yours."

I handed him a ten. Added a five.

Of course, this irked me. Impossible, I thought, that anyone would travel anywhere, especially on an interstate, without money for tolls. He grinned and expected me to bail him out, like a little kid. What if we hadn't met up en route? Did he think of that? There wasn't anything for me to do except practice from A.A. "Let go, let God." I was still annoyed.

Barnes, Sagamore, Philadelphia, and I arrived at the motel at 5:00 PM, in time for the animals to play and jump on and off the bed—making it impossible for me to nap—and to have a leisurely bath before dinner. Francis got lost and showed up at 8:00 PM.

"Ha, ha, I've always had a lousy sense of direction, you know, hon?"

I was too tired to laugh.

The next day, when we arrived in North Carolina, we found out the moving truck was delayed. While we waited and had a few leisurely days at the Residence Inn in Durham, Francis learned that a large commission he was counting on had fallen through. He was sorry, he told me, but he had no available cash and would not be able to pay the $4,000 cost of the move. I was speechless.

"I never kited a check before," he said. "There's no money behind the check I wrote for the movers."

While Francis was away doing errands the head Mayflower mover put the receipts for our belongings in my hands. I signed and now I was about to be minus a hefty chunk of cash. The financial situation manifesting itself was new to me. At first, I was not overly concerned. We had always traveled and dined upscale on Francis's dime, on his credit cards. We both worked on commission, and were familiar with fluctuations in money supply. In our courting days, we had discussed finances and the expected settlement Francis would receive when his divorce was final. Was it only my assumption—and a big one at that—that Francis would be entitled to half the value of his home? Where were his back-up funds?

I was too tired to cry.

The house we were renting in Carrboro was pricey and too big for us, but the physician homeowner needed to move on to his new job in Baltimore, and was willing to accept our pets. A wooded area in back was a fertile hunting ground for the kittens. There were nice paths for walks and a brook for Barnes to splash in. It was a simple ten-minute drive to Chapel Hill and not much more to Durham.

Along with being a willing helper, Francis was handy. He cheerfully swept the floor, hung pictures, lugged furniture from spot to spot, hugged me often. He spurted, "I love you, hon," when I least expected it, as we were shining up the rosy future, moving forward with the dream.

Then after we'd settled in a bit, a phone call from Francis. "Silly," he said. "Losing the car is silly. Can you come to the library and help me find it and we can have lunch in Chapel Hill?" Francis went to the library for a portion of every day to do research on employment opportunities.

"We had lunch before you left, my love, but Barnes and I will be right along."

Later that afternoon, Francis settled into the sofa with a Diet Pepsi and asked if I knew when we started classes.

"Well, Francis," I said as I looked up from the cardboard box I was unpacking, "you need a job, right?"

Surely he was kidding about classes, wasn't he? Did he think he was a student again? His question miffed me. And why the hell did he keep getting lost every time he drove farther than the center of Chapel Hill, which was just a few miles up the road?

I drove him to the few interviews that materialized in Raleigh and in Cary to be sure he got there. None of these opportunities worked out. Either Francis didn't want the job or the executive search firm did not offer him a position. Appointments were delayed. Hot prospects had gone out of business. Contacts had moved. I got a part-time job at a new housing development and fought to keep the nagging, something-is-wrong thoughts on the back burner, day after day.

Of course, I rationalized it must be me, something I just didn't understand. Perhaps it just takes time to find employment in the executive search field. Francis was his cheerful self and did not appear at all concerned about not being able to find employment. It was just a temporary stall, I told myself, again and again. I believed in my Francis.

Months slid along, vacation-like. We took day trips to explore North Carolina, walked, talked, held hands, played fetch with Barnes. Smiled. Waited. Waited.

Finally, in the beginning of September, Francis had a date for his most promising interview. He looked very spiffy when he set out at 8:00 AM. for his 10:00 AM. appointment in the University Towers, an eyesore skyscraper that could be seen for miles around, near South Square in Durham. We had done trial runs and I mapped out directions and taped them to his dashboard, just in case he needed help. After doing some errands, I returned home at around 11:00 AM. A lump sprung into my gut when I saw Francis's car in the driveway. I found him. In bed, under the covers, in his suit. Asleep.

"I couldn't find the place, hon. Couldn't do it."

"Why, Francis? After all our trial runs, how come, what happened?"

"I called them and said my car broke down. I'll reschedule."

That was the last of the promising interviews.

Of course, I was upset, confused, and worried. I counseled myself to be patient, to hold onto the thread that things would work out. What else was there to do? Just hold on. It was frightening to dig beneath the surface and even worse to see Francis so blasé about our situation.

*   *   *

In the fall, I went to visit Peter and his family in Vermont for a few days. I phoned Francis and reminded him Barnes and I would be arriving at Raleigh-Durham Airport at 7:00 PM. Francis assured me he would be there to meet us, he had missed us, he loved me. I couldn't wait to see him. Would he bring a red rose?

Francis was not at the airport. I called home. No answer. I had him paged at the airport. Once. Again. No response. Taxis weren't big enough to take Barnes, his pet porter, and me to Carrboro. We waited hours for a van to show up and drive us home. I woke Francis. Asked him. "Why? What happened? Where were you?"

"I went. You weren't there."

"But I was there. What happened?"

"I don't know, hon. I don't know."

All that he could tell me was that he went to the airport after I had called, around two o'clock, couldn't find me so he went home. He'd had hot dogs and beans with our neighbor, William.

"I went, hon. You weren't there."

"Of course, I was there."

"I went. I was there, hon."

"When did you go, Francis?"

"Two o'clock, hon, and you were not there."

"Right, Francis. I was not there at 2:00 PM. We arrived, on time, as scheduled, at 7:00 PM."

A note was on my pillow—"Sleep tight. I love you. See you in the morning, sweetheart. I love you." How could I possibly sleep? What in God's name was happening? How could Francis possibly sleep?

It was hard to stay mad at Francis for any length of time despite his seemingly senseless behavior. So much was good about us. Wide awake in the darkness, my knees pulled close to my chest, I relived the falling-in-love days, the hours walking on beaches and talking about places we'd been and places we'd like to go; the bagels; the truck stops; the elegant, tiny confections on crystal and silver trays at the Helmsley. Our giddy, singing-in-the-rain kind of love.

A little giggle surprised me as I remembered shopping for a Christmas present with Francis, back in 1992. Now it seemed like another lifetime. I had gotten off the bus and tried not to stare at the lumps of homeless people curled up against the recently white-washed walls of the Port Authority.

"Hey, bootiful," I'd heard and I knew it was my Francis, playfully imitating a New Jersey accent, as he briskly walked toward me, wearing his heavy black chesterfield coat with the black velvet collar.

We'd hugged. Long. Tight. Our hands clasped. On the street in Times Square, I stuck my tongue out to catch a floppy snowflake. Like a delicate meringue, it melted before I could savor it. The grime and dirt of New York City was being shrouded in a soft snow. Blaring taxi horns and street noises were pierced by tinkling bells rung by the Salvation Army Santa Clauses. Aromas of roasting chestnuts and grilling sausages tempted a passerby. Strangers nodded at each other, happy to see the gigantic Douglas fir safely installed on its lofty throne in Rockefeller Plaza.

We had ambled into the Godiva Chocolate Shop for a whiff and two little pieces of bliss on our way to an expensive boutique on Fifth Avenue. I had never been clothes shopping with a man before. It felt odd.

Once there, Francis had coaxed me: "Please put this on."

Out of habit, I had glanced at the price tag and shuddered.

"Gorgeous," he'd exclaimed when I modeled the classic knee-length silk suit, hot pink with gold buttons, pleated skirt, size two. Francis admired my legs, uttered a clicking sound.

"Please wrap this for my lady," he had told the clerk and dug into his left hand pants pocket for his wad of credit cards, cash, and pink memo slips. We'd then gone to Brooks Brothers. Francis bought his standard button-down shirts, light blue, white, 17 1/2 neck, 33-inch sleeve, and a large, square, red and green floral silk scarf to brighten my classic black winter coat.

"It's you, my love. It's you."

I had felt like a princess and hadn't been able to stop grinning.

Despite the lunchtime crowd in a deli-bagel den, we had managed to get a window seat. As Francis shook down two packets of Sweet N' Low, he'd asked, "Do you know much about sex?"

What could I have possibly said? "Oh, yes, sure I do. Oh, no, I am afraid not. Oh, well, a little of this and that, you know, maybe." I'd taken as big a bite of my bagel as possible. Before I had to answer the question, Francis had spoken. He proposed that we walk up the avenue to Barnes and Noble to get a little reference material.

"Really?" I'd asked.

"Really," he'd said.

We had pushed through the revolving door at Barnes and Noble.

I'd headed straight to the yoga and meditation section, stood still, and stared at the bookshelf. I'd wanted to run back to the street, but I'd joined Francis, a tome under his arm, in the checkout line.

"Do you think your brother will like his birthday present?" I'd asked in a too-loud, too-obvious voice as Francis had offered up the book and fished for a credit card.

Later, we had sat with thighs touching on a pink-and-mauve striped love seat in the privacy of a Victorian bed and breakfast at the Jersey Shore and peeled off the black and green swirl gift-wrap with the reverence of opening an heirloom Bible. In our generation, at least for me, sex was not something to experiment with or to openly discuss.

"Well. Look at that. Would you like to try that?" Francis had inquired with the naïveté of a five-year-old boy suggesting I pull down my underpants if he'd pull down his.

In the morning, despite the December chill, Francis had used a dime to laboriously carve our initials with a heart on the railing of the Spring Lake Bridge. I was quite cold and moved from foot to foot to resist shivering. He was totally engrossed in the project; I couldn't suggest he speed it up. On our ride back to Allendale after breakfast, we'd held hands, letting go only when Francis had to shift Bup's gears.

Francis never uttered another word about the airport fiasco. He cheerfully gave Barnes belly rubs, smiled at me, and offered to get me cups of coffee. How he could mess up the simple plan to pick us up baffled me. I stayed angry too long, until finally I was able to let it go, as we had learned in A.A.

Several months later, I was delighted to see Francis walking toward me at the airport gate after another trip to Vermont. He was carrying an umbrella, two hardcover books, and three newspapers.

"My God, Francis, how long have you been here?"

"Oh, overnight. For days. But I don't know where the car is," he said as we walked into each other for a hug and a smooch. "But, I don't know, don't know where the car is," he said again. And again. I tossed his comment off, not wanting to believe him. Surely he could find the car. There was a parking lot right next to the airline terminal, for easy pick-up access. I was relieved that he had managed to get to the airport, but I didn't understand the raincoat and umbrella since it was a clear evening and there was a covered walkway from the parking lot to the terminal.

We got the luggage and sprung Barnes out of his pet porter and walked up and down the parking lot aisles for over an hour. Nothing gave Francis a clue as to where the car was. Then he mentioned trees. I couldn't find one tree. We spent another hour searching and then, again, I paid for a van to take us home. When we got to our driveway, Francis hurried into the house and returned with seventy-three cents to help defray the $35 cost of the van.

Of course, I was exhausted, but not too tired to be very worried about what was going on with Francis. Getting lost and forgetting things had become commonplace and now it appeared that his reasoning power, at least some of his reasoning power, had disappeared. I had to work hard to cobble together possible reasons for his behavior. What the hell was going on?

The Raleigh-Durham Airport Tracer of Lost Cars Division located the car within a half hour the next afternoon. Bup was in a long-term parking lot with plenty of trees. And indeed, it had rained early in the morning when Francis had set out for the airport. A red rose, beautiful and droopy, was waiting for me on the passenger seat.

I put as much of this turmoil as possible aside, tucked it away inside, and went to the market, alone. Driving home, it flashed into my head that maybe Francis had Alzheimer's disease, a condition I knew next to nothing about but had seen mentioned in the press. It had something to do with forgetfulness. Maybe it applied to my

Francis. What would the treatment be?

"I'm just in love!" was Francis's cheerful, stock reply whenever we talked about plans that were forgotten, dates that were confused. Even after the worn, beige L.L. Bean bag that never left his side had gone missing and he wasn't bothered. Now I knew he needed a doctor's appointment, an evaluation. How could I tell him this? Suggesting an evaluation implied there was something wrong with him and, yes, there certainly was, but did he know it? We were always up front with each other and open with our thoughts, so as soon as I came home from the market, I walked in the door and, finding Francis sitting by the sunny window in the kitchen, I blurted out: "We need a doctor's appointment for you."

He surprised me by readily agreeing. But his reaction was affectless. "That's a good idea. Do you want a Diet Pepsi, hon?" he said.

Of course, I was struggling not to be overwhelmed. I repeated the serenity prayer: "God, grant me the serenity to accept the things I cannot change; courage to change the things I can; and wisdom to know the difference." Said it constantly. One day at a time was the only way to handle what was happening. More like one hour, one minute at a time. I had been in turmoil before. I would be okay. Francis was calm, along for the ride. Where, oh, where, was the Francis I fell in love with? It was better for me not to wonder, not to think.

The very next morning, eleven months after we had arrived in North Carolina, we went to the Family Doctor Walk-In Clinic located in an upscale mini-mall in Chapel Hill. Birds chirped in the budding pear trees that lined the sidewalks. The office was bright and cheerful and stocked with magazines—*People, Golf, Newsweek, Ranger Rick*. It was a Monday morning, late April. Francis had an appointment with Dr. Anne Varren who administered part of the standard tests for Alzheimer's. She asked Francis questions like what county are you in? Francis didn't know. What building is this? Francis didn't know. What is today's date? Francis grinned and looked over at me for the answer. The current season? Francis didn't know.

I tried to appear calm, but I was astounded. I suspected that Dr. Varren saw through my bravado. She was reassuring, very caring and gentle. She explained that she was not a specialist and that the probable diagnosis of Alzheimer's was made only after all other causes of dementia were ruled out.

Of course, I hated the word dementia. Damn. What a horrible word dementia is. Don't let me hear that. For God's sake, don't let Francis hear that.

Francis was to have blood work done to rule out a deficiency in vitamin b and an MRI to rule out a tumor. A cancellation at Durham Regional Hospital meant we could go for the MRI that afternoon. We had time for lunch in Chapel Hill, and Francis could have his favorite Brunswick stew at Mama Dip's Kitchen while I struggled over so many choices of real southern cooking.

Later, Francis had an appointment with Dr. Gurtel, an Alzheimer's specialist, in addition to being a neurologist and a psychologist, at Durham Regional Hospital. Thunderstorms had been predicted and they arrived, booming and clapping as we drove out of our driveway at six thirty that morning, coffee mugs by our sides, and Barnes curled up on the backseat. Dr. Gurtel, a warm, pleasant-looking, middle-aged man, informed us that Francis's MRI was normal, as was his blood work. He asked me to leave the room so that additional tests could be administered. When I was invited back into the office, Dr. Gurtel explained that Francis most probably had Alzheimer's disease.

Oh, what a relief, I thought. My shoulders noticeably relaxed and dropped down from up by my ears where I had been hauling them around. Now, at last we could fix things,

"What can we do, Doctor? How do we cure that?"

"There is no cure," Dr. Gurtel said.

He gently explained, "There are methods of slowing the disease but there is no cure at this time. The good news is that with all the research being done, perhaps we will have a cure soon. Go see Dr. Eveymore, a primary care physician in Chapel Hill, whom I think you will like, for a complete physical and return in a couple of weeks for further discussion. Bring any questions you might have."

We didn't know enough about the disease to have questions.

Francis tucked his hand in mine as we left the hospital and we walked in step out into the storm.

Of course, neither one of us had the slightest idea what this would mean, how it would affect our life together, what the future now held, or how we would deal with it. What I did know, in the deepest crevice of my gut, was that I would do what had to be done to keep us safe. For as long as I could. That's what you do when you love someone.

Do the next best thing

We returned to Dr. Gurtel after the physical exam, which had gone well. He explained that a drug called Cognex might slow the symptoms. Francis would have to have weekly blood tests for a month or more to monitor the drug's level and its side effects.

"It's your choice, Francis," I said.

"Let's try it," he said.

We left the doctor's office and headed home, in silence. It was the first time that Francis didn't suggest we stop in Chapel Hill for lunch.

Dr. Gurtel had agreed to mail us a statement with Francis's diagnosis of "probable Alzheimer's." We learned that a positive diagnosis could only be made by examining the brain after death. I helped Francis send notes with copies of his probable diagnosis to Mattie and his children and expected there would be immediate phone calls or at least letters in response. What there was was nothing. Nada. Until two weeks later when a letter arrived from Mattie. Francis shook his head as he read. He gave the letter to me. Mattie wrote that she had done research and asked around and there was no diagnosis for Alzheimer's. She added that Joby (her nickname for Francis) was a strong man and he should not let the doctors tell him he had Alzheimer's. I was shocked and could not imagine why she would argue against the doctor's diagnosis or, worse yet, advise that it be ignored. It was not my style to badmouth any of Francis's family, but it was tough to be silent this time. The letter appeared to bother me more than it bothered Francis.

I read what I could find about the mysterious and baffling Alzheimer's disease. The information in books like *The Thirty-Six Hour Day* was overwhelming and very depressing, to put it mildly, and I struggled, not wanting to believe what I read. I learned that Alzheimer's patients could just slip away, lose all of their mental skills, all deductive reasoning, and regress to childhood, to babyhood and total dependency, yet still be alive. The multiple and diverse symptoms were uncountable. An Alzheimer's patient could be expected to forget things, particularly recently learned material, and would have difficulty accomplishing normal day-to-day living tasks, such as setting a table. When Francis could not locate a simple word, he described the activity. For example, a comb would become the thing you put on your hair. There might be disorientation with time and place and confusion with dates, with past and present. Increased sleeping, poor judgment, personality changes, dependency and forgetting friends and family were symptoms of the disease.

Of course, in looking back I see that over time these symptoms had manifested themselves in Francis. Sometimes when I asked Francis what he wanted to do he grinned and responded "I just wanna be with you." How sweet, I'd thought. In reality, he likely could not think of what he wanted to do.

What would Cognex do? I wondered if it could make Francis feel more comfortable and capable in daily living. Or would it just prolong the agony of what was to come? Was it worth the gamble?

At any rate, it was Francis's decision and he opted to try the medication. Research indicated that of all the people who have Alzheimer's disease, only about 5 percent, or approximately 200,000 people, have symptoms before they are sixty-five years old, which is categorized as early onset Alzheimer's. The hypothesis that early onset Alzheimer's progressed more quickly was not backed up by hard data. There was some indication that the disease was hereditary and I couldn't help but feel this must be terrifying for Francis's children. Some research suggested that the disease starts many years—at least ten—before any symptoms manifest themselves. If Francis had any memory problems in his younger days, I surmised it was passed off as part of his excessive drinking. In my personal experience, during my drinking years there were periods of forgetfulness—painful experiences I tried to ignore.

We talked about the future. It was easy to talk about it because we had no idea what would come. The only consistency in the manifestation of Alzheimer's seemed to be its inconsistency, its unpredictability, and the swings from seeming rational to being clueless.

Soon after Francis's diagnosis, his divorce was finalized. The exact date has left my memory and was overshadowed by a giant revelation. Along with the settlement papers came the announcement that back real estate taxes were due on his marital house and that he had amassed large credit card debts totaling close to $200,000 and therefore would not be receiving any reimbursement from his divorce settlement. I was flabbergasted. Struck dumb. He had never hinted at any debt when we discussed finances before we'd leapt into life together and moved to North Carolina. We had always dined and traveled upscale on Francis's dime. Or plastic.

Of course, it eventually dawned on me that, by this date, he didn't understand his debts or how they had accumulated. Worse was the fact that he didn't appear to care.

Within a few weeks of beginning to take Cognex, Francis noticeably changed. The drug lessened his confusion, improved his awareness, and generally made him more comfortable.

In the midst of this, we had to pack up again and look for a place to live because our lease was due to expire. The packing process went smoothly. Francis cheerfully did the things I asked him to do. Giving him concrete structure was good for both of us. The most difficulty he had was making decisions and initiating actions.

In the process of packing, we unearthed his L.L. Bean bag, which I had tucked into a blanket chest for safekeeping, and had subsequently forgotten. Finding it reminded me that Francis had never seemed worried about its disappearance. In fact, he rarely worried about anything anymore. I began to see his lack of worry as a small blessing of the disease.

We opened the Bean bag together and revealed its contents: a stash of long outdated and mostly unopened bills and communications from credit card companies requesting payment, offering payment plans, threatening legal action. All addressed to his former New Jersey address.

I can't remember what, if anything, Francis said, or what, if anything, I said. Genuine surprise registered on his face. I was dumbstruck.

Of course, it didn't occur to me that Francis might have been hiding these bills from his family. Nor did I know how long the practice had been going on. Never did I entertain the notion that he would willfully deceive me.

House-hunting together was pleasant. I assumed that Francis's self-confidence was taking a big beating from Alzheimer's, so I made a point of asking his opinions about the neighborhoods and the houses we saw. Most of the time he echoed me, but he vetoed my first-choice house because it had too steep a driveway, a feature I hadn't noticed. In a short time, we found a cute, small cape. It was under construction, so I could customize it by combining two of the small upstairs bedrooms into the kind of spacious master bedroom I'd always desired. The house was on a cul-de-sac, had a sunlit back deck overlooking a large wooded area, was close to shopping in Durham, and was within easy walking distance to a leash-free dog park for Barnes. Eleven Willow Brook suited us just fine.

We were moving into our new home. On moving day, Ronald phoned and said that he and his wife, Lisa, were in the area and could come by. Francis and I were exhausted from the moving activities and not in good form for a surprise visit. I figured they would prefer to have some private time so I stayed home and unpacked and sent them out to dinner.

When I put our new address and phone number in Francis's pocket, Ronald said, "I can't believe you don't know how to get home, Dad."

They left and returned home more quickly than a leisurely dinner should take at the Outback Steakhouse. Lisa brought me an uneaten steak and a ruptured baked potato, then squatted on the floor to play with Barnes while we watched, quietly. I wondered if Ronald saw how withdrawn Francis had become. Who knew when the disease had started crippling his brain? The man Ronald called Dad, the jovial and outgoing man who had fascinated me in the late 1980s, was disappearing.

Ronald sent a letter after his brief visit suggesting to his dad that he "change your life style, contact your old friends, be someone worth remembering." Francis shook his head as he read.

Of course, I did not know about the previous relationship between Ronald and Francis, but I found Ronald's letter appalling. Perhaps I unfairly blamed the children for the rifts and lack of communication. I saw things from their father's point of view and hated to see him hurt. Naïve as it may have been, I had expected a companionable relation-

ship with Francis's children. In my mind, divorce from a spouse did not include divorce from one's children.

It was an additional eighteen months before I clearly understood that I could not help Francis reconcile with his children.

"I give up," I said. "Your issues with your kids are yours."

Francis surprised me by saying, "Right you are." He seemed relieved that I was butting out. I guessed his disease was claiming more of his unsolvable issues and I hoped that was some relief for him.

Surprisingly, a job for Francis in a recruiting firm in Cary, North Carolina, materialized shortly after the diagnosis. I reasoned that Francis was familiar with the field and fervently wished that this would work out, not only for the money, but also to help him feel that he was doing something worthwhile. Francis had a tough time handling the forty-five minute drive to the office and told me he took a different route every day. I asked him to drive us to his office one morning and saw for myself how he forgot where to go and where he had been. He laughed it off, reminding me of his poor sense of direction. Rather than worry about him wandering and getting lost, I led him in to work in the morning and met him at the end of the day and he followed me home.

By the third week on the job, Francis started complaining that his boss didn't know how to do anything right or how to be productive. For more than ten years, Francis had been a successful vice president in two recruiting firms in competitive New York City. His job in Cary doing cold-call telephone work, nine to five, had to be demoralizing. I urged Francis to try to make it work, but at the end of the month he handed me his check for the trial period. Trial period? He had not mentioned that was what it had been.

Of course, I thought about why Francis didn't tell me the details of his job or complain about how frequently he got lost. Was he embarrassed about his ineptitude or did he simply forget? If he forgot, did it bother him?

Did I notice that I had stopped asking questions when I was afraid of the answers and that our communication was slipping away? Did that register at all with me? Of course not. I didn't want it to register.

Another phone call from Francis. "This is big time lost. Big time."

He was calling from Brightleaf Square, a small shopping center in downtown Durham. His frustration came across loud and clear about his lost car.

"I'm retiring the car," he added.

Music to my ears. I had read about the problems that went along with getting an Alzheimer patient to surrender the car. A car was a gateway to freedom, but Francis's driving had become frightfully dangerous. He ran stop signs and slowed down at green lights, sometimes stopping altogether. There had to be a God watching out for drivers like him. My days of riding with him were over, but I hadn't known how to suggest he quit driving altogether. And now he'd done it himself.

Francis's car, Bup, held many memories for us, including when we got caught in a policeman's flashlight beam in a restaurant parking lot while we were making out like high schoolers. And Bup would always travel on a snow day. We would play hooky from work and go to the movies. Off we would sail in Bup, skidding, sliding, laughing, loving winter, loving being together, loving a snow day.

But more recent memories weren't so carefree. One Sunday morning, we had gone out for a shrimp-and-grits brunch at our favorite Chapel Hill restaurant, Crook's Corner, before I went to work. He was to follow me in his car along a sleepy, tree-lined residential street. I had been wearing the black felt hat Francis had bought for me in Georgetown and when I glanced in my rearview mirror to adjust the tilt of the brim, I had seen Francis swinging a very wide—too wide—U-turn, and heading back towards home, driving south in the northbound lane. As soon as I could, I'd turned my car around to catch up with him and found him pulled over on a side street, opening to the puzzle page of the newspaper that never left his side. "Hi, hon. We going somewhere today?" What was there to do but smile at my loveable Francis and be thankful he was safe?

At Brightleaf Square, Francis was standing right where he said he would be. We found the car and straight away took it for an appraisal. I didn't want to miss this opportunity. We wrote a for-sale sign, advertised in the local paper, cleaned out the glove box and the trunk. The second person who looked at it bought it with cash. Francis handed the six hundred and fifty dollars to me and said, "How about a trip to the sea?"

Two weeks later, we were packing to go to a duplex rental on Emerald Isle, North Carolina. One block from the sea, the house was perfect. It was cheerfully furnished with inviting sofas, lots of pillows, and a rocking chair by the huge picture window. All of the kitchen appliances were modern and it had a washer and dryer in the garage next to the pile of beach chairs, shovels, pails, and the charcoal for the grill. We rigged up a divider barricade with upturned chairs on the front deck to keep Barnes on our side, but the duplex neighbors frequently invited him over for a bone. The weather was spectacular. Every day we played at the beach, cooked out, or explored the island. The water was too cold for me, but dear Francis took Barnes into the ocean and taught him how to ride the waves. Barnes grinned as he returned to the beach, rolled in the sand, and quickly pranced back into the water, his otter-like tail slapping the salty air. He even learned to retrieve a ball thrown over the waves' breaking point. People who walked by stopped to watch and clap, and I cheered for my dog, cheered for my man. On our walks at the edge of the sea, Francis picked up seashells and later wrote in the shells "I love you," a message that never faded.

Francis's unpaid medical bills were piling up. It was clear he needed some sort of financial aid. It was also clear he wasn't going to do anything about it. I could, though, and would.

The first appointment was at the Medicare office in Raleigh. After tedious interviews and mountainous paperwork, Francis became eligible for Medicare, which took care of his medical bills, and he was granted early Social Security. He was referred to Social Services in Durham to apply for financial aid, which sounded nicer than "disability." We headed into the bowels of Durham to the Social Services office. Francis looked jaunty in his white ducks and blue button-down Brooks Brothers shirt with the sleeves rolled up. I was wearing a floral wrap skirt from Talbots. It was a beautiful, cloudless morning. Social Services was in a renovated but grungy, old, brick tobacco warehouse. The crowded parking lot was littered with McDonald's wrappers, soda bottles, empty cigarette packs and butts. It didn't get much better on the inside.

We located two metal folding chairs next to each other in the waiting room, which was packed with young mothers, some of them very pregnant with toddlers clinging to their feet, and elderly, forlorn men and women. Some looked homeless. They all looked hungry. I could tell that people wondered what we were there for, clean and dressed as if we were dashing off to a lawn party by the river. It made me uncomfortable. I tried not to fidget or make eye contact.

Francis had psychiatric examinations and an interview, which I was not allowed to attend, to determine if he qualified for disability. The answer was no. Disability denied at this time. Although Francis could not work in his given field, he was deemed employable.

A merry-go-round of searching for suitable employment began. Francis went to the nearby Harris-Teeter market to apply for a job and then, at my urging, returned a few times to check on the status of his application. Later, I found the application crumpled up in a wastebasket. The simple form must have been too difficult for him to fill out and he didn't think or was too embarrassed to ask for my help.

In a few weeks, we discovered a job that sounded good: sweeping up and putting away chairs after meetings at a nearby church. There were a few initial visits which seemed to go well. However, the pastor dismissed Francis when he learned we were living together but were not married, siblings, or mother and son. Mother and son? Was that remotely believable?

Finally, a job was available at Rose's, a variety store in a small mall that Francis could walk to. At that point, I took a short trip to Vermont.

When I returned home, Francis said, "Come on and shop at Rose's. I get a discount."

We filled up a shopping cart with all sorts of maybe useful and maybe necessary items.

At the checkout counter, the teenage clerk said, "He don't work here no more."

Francis shrugged his shoulders and I bought the stuff anyway. Immediately, I went to see his supervisor. She told me Francis didn't stock the shelves like he was instructed to do, sat in the break room in a snit, borrowed money for the soda machine, and was rude. This was not a Francis I had ever heard of. When I explained that Francis had Alzheimer's, the supervisor said she wished she had known that. It was a fact I did not even think about disclosing. But he couldn't stock shelves if he couldn't find the correct aisle for the merchandise. How humiliating and frustrating for him. He'd never mentioned any difficulties.

Of course, my tendency was to assume he was capable of taking care of things at his own pace. Perhaps I should have intervened more, but how much and when? I had only my gut for guidance and I felt it was important to foster Francis's independence and capabilities.

During the following months, Francis's behavior changed markedly. For the first time, I described him as "moody" in my journal. He snapped at me when I asked him simple questions. Additionally, his motor coordination deteriorated and he frequently spilled things or dribbled the coffee he was drinking on his shirt. He forgot how to load and start the dishwasher.

We returned to the Social Security office and reapplied for disability. I helped Francis with the intricate application. Months later he began receiving checks based on his years in the work force. He was fifty-seven-and-a-half-years old. In the prime of his life, some would say.

Although attempts to find employment had failed, there was a temporary solution that kept Francis engaged. Everybody loved him at the Senior Citizen Center in Chapel Hill where he volunteered setting up tables, cleaning the kitchen sink, doing odd jobs and sweeping, sweeping, sweeping. He liked being part of the busy activity and seemed happy. It was a big relief for me to know that the staff was keeping an eye on him and I had some time to recharge.

Every six months, Francis was required to take the same Alzheimer's test again. I was shocked as I learned that reality was out of reach for him. He failed to identify the day, the month, and the town he was in. I felt embarrassed for my Francis. He looked about the same as when I'd met him, with less hair on the top of his head, but his beautiful, longer silver fringe was still attractive. Maybe he had gained a few pounds. On closer examination, though, his eyes and his mannerisms revealed that something was different. In the doctor's office one day, he shifted his focus, turned his head. What was he looking for? What was he trying to get away from?

Dr. Eveymore sensed that Francis was getting agitated. He treated Francis like an important adult and gently explained, "This is all expendable knowledge, isn't it? With all the research that is going on, we have reason to hope for some therapy that will ease your situation."

It was a miniscule thread of hope to cling to.

We drove home. I made a pot of coffee, put Fig Newtons on an antique pewter plate, sat at the kitchen table, and asked Francis to bring me a cup of coffee. He brought just the pot, sat down, smiled. I closed my eyes briefly, returned his smile, and got up to fetch two cups.

Early in the afternoon the next day, I walked in the door of the senior center and Robin, the supervisor, asked me to come upstairs to her office. "We all love Francis," she started, "but his increased confusion has made it impossible for him to follow directions. We can no longer have him here."

I was disappointed with the news, but I had expected it sooner or later. I found Francis in the kitchen, meticulously wiping out the double stainless sinks with a miniscule piece of paper towel. He flashed me his special I-am-so-happy-to-see-you grin, and came over to take my hand.

"Barnes is with me and he's invited you to come out for ice cream with us, okay?" I said as we closed the door to the senior center.

That evening I asked, "How about a shower, Francis?"

"I just had a shower, hon."

"Two days ago, Francis. Do you want to be smelly?"

Here was the same guy who had wanted to jump into the shower or a bubble bath together any time of day or night. This time he clenched his teeth and looked mean.

Of course, I shouldn't have asked if he wanted to be smelly. He probably didn't notice, didn't care. What's to smell? No exercise, no sex, no sweat. And did the act of undressing make him feel vulnerable? It occurred to me that many children go through periods of extreme modesty. Maybe that's why he wore extra shirts and sweaters on top of one another. Analyzing was tiring for me. Exhausting.

One morning, I returned from a walk with Barnes and smelled heat as I opened the front door. All four burners on the stove were on full blast. I shut them off and pointed out how dangerous it was to do something like that.

Francis replied, "I'd better stay away from the kitchen, hon." A perfectly rational response. He still looked normal, so wonderful on the outside. It was hard to imagine the confusion that must be roiling on his insides.

Francis's symptoms slowly became more numerous and obvious. In early September 1996, we returned home from a long afternoon at Jordan Lake with Barnes.

The boat launching area had been flooded in the aftermath of Hurricane Bonnie and kids, dogs, adults were milling around, glad to be out of the house. Barnes, always the social chairman, greeted every human and every dog, stood at alert, watched the launching boats, and swam out to greet each new boat as it came ashore. Francis got in the swing of things, took off his shoes and socks, went wading and threw tennis balls for any dog that would fetch. Everyone exchanged stories of how they coped with being without electricity and water for four or more days.

That evening as I was fixing supper, Francis asked, "Why do you suppose Barnes is so tired?"

I was dismayed. He did not remember a single thing about our afternoon. I could no longer rationalize that the forgetting was a temporary or occasional problem.

Of course, my Francis was gradually becoming a different person, but I did not see it. He was annoyingly casual about critical things, like leaving the burners on, and lovingly playful about giving me a smooch. We were deeply connected. Were there things I should have, would have, could have done had I known better?

Duke University sponsored a monthly joint patient-caregiver Alzheimer's support group. Francis was willing to give it a try. We were late arriving. A large group, male and female, patient and caregiver, was assembled in a circle. The leaders welcomed us graciously, got us nametags, and rustled up two chairs.

Francis whispered to me, "These people are so old! We're the youngest, by ten or fifteen years." He was right; we were a good deal younger.

Without warning, a patient started rambling in a loud voice, repeating phrases, and uttering gibberish. The tension and agitation in the group increased noticeably. Soon, the patients went off to a separate room. Francis was reluctant to leave my side, but a skilled leader stepped in to guide him along.

The general topic in the caregivers group was behavioral problems. A man reported that his wife had been putting her clothes on inside out or backwards.

"So what? What difference does it really make?" a caregiver interjected and the group agreed it was no big deal.

Sundowning—when the patient does not know the caregiver at the end of the day—was discussed at length. We talked about difficulties encountered when patients no longer know family members and when long-time friends gradually stop visiting and drift out of touch. A weepy caregiver shared that she felt she was giving up her own life and was living the life of her Alzheimer's-afflicted husband. Many heads nodded in knowing agreement.

Given the unpredictable behavior of Alzheimer's patients, it was easier to avoid being in public situations. Clearly, I was not alone in noting that the world Francis and I lived in had become very small and isolated. We went for walks with Barnes, shopped at the supermarket, showed up at A.A. meetings, went to bed early. In the other world, the big world, news was happening. The scandal involving President Clinton and Monica Lewinsky was breaking into the national media. The Lunar Prospector was launched to survey the moon's surface. Tiger Woods had claimed the 1999 PGA Player of the Year, the Arnold Palmer Award, the Jack Nicklaus Trophy, and the Byron Nelson and Vardon Trophy awards. Out there, business as usual.

A patient in the other room hollered, ran down the hall and out the front door toward the parking lot. His ever-vigilant caregiver bolted from our group to get him back. I had read about frightening and depressing occurrences that were likely to happen to Alzheimer's patients. It came much closer to home when I heard group members tell of their problematic personal experiences, when their patients showed up in public naked, insulted friends and strangers, or suddenly became very angry and uncooperative.

Of course, it bothered me to hear griping and negative comments like, "Just wait and you will see," or "In time, it will most likely happen." I noted that the patients at this group meeting were much more advanced than Francis. Their caregivers could well be suffering from burnout. Quietly, I vowed to work very hard at staying upbeat and being supportive of Francis.

I met Francis in the hallway after the meeting and asked how it went for him. He just shook his head and looked down at his shoes. We were invited to join the group for lunch at a Chinese restaurant around the corner. An authoritative caregiver was concerned we would get lost and insisted we ride with him and his wife. Perhaps I looked more overwhelmed than I thought. Francis never left my side at the restaurant and I clung close to the leaders. It was a strain. The caregivers tried to be relaxed, but it didn't work very well, and one could not help but notice the vacant, blank expressions on the Alzheimer's patients' faces, their rigidity, and their sense of emptiness. The arrival of the fortune cookies was a blessed relief.

Shortly after we got home, Francis went off to the hardware store, a mile down the road. He was gone for two hours. Usually, when he was delayed or lost he would call me and I would give him directions or meet him. This time he didn't call. I sat and stared at the phone. Finally, I called the police who arrived at the front door about the same time Francis strolled in the back door. They had a laugh about that. I was not laughing.

We traveled together to Vermont frequently after it became apparent that Francis could not be left home unsupervised. Time with my family was a required tonic for me. We were also naturally isolated at the Jeffersonville house and it was easy to be there with Francis. We were masters at hanging out together. Barnes chased squirrels in the summer and burrowed in the snow in the winter. Francis swept in the summer, shoveled in the winter. I enjoyed rave reviews for my experimental creative cooking no matter what the result.

On Francis's sixty-second birthday we met Peter at a café. Francis managed to order and pay for our coffees. Peter and I sat in a booth and watched as Francis put sugar into Peter's black coffee. Francis denied adding it. Peter nodded to me to confirm sugar. It was an important moment of unspoken understanding between Peter and me as we acknowledged that Francis was disconnected from his own behavior. Henceforth, communication with Peter became easier and I felt increased support from him.

The birthday gifts of chocolate bars pleased Francis immensely. He opened up a bar and offered us the first pieces of dark chocolate.

"Pretty good for a three-year-old, huh," Francis said when he saw that my grandson, Connor had signed a card and added hugs and kisses.

On the way home, we stopped at the supermarket. I was in the checkout lane and had forgotten to get cat food and asked Francis to go and get it. He returned with dog food, and on the next attempt, with kitty litter. When we got in the car he cried and would only say that he would be all right.

"Please don't shut me out, Francis."

"I won't," he said in a tiny voice.

Of course, I felt shut out. What did "all right" mean to Francis? Our verbal communication was slipping away, fast. Our nonverbal commu-

nication, though, remained steadfast.

One evening at dinnertime at Peter's house, Amy was busy at the stove and, to be helpful, I handed a bunch of napkins to Francis to distribute around the table. Francis went to the dining room, but was confused about what to do next.

Peter was standing nearby, turned toward me and whispered, "He doesn't know what to do, Mom." Peter sounded incredulous, but I saw that he more fully understood the circumstances Francis and I were experiencing even more. "I'll help you, Francis," Peter said.

Peter and Amy phoned us after we had returned to Durham and asked if we could come up in March and care for Connor, so they might travel to London for a week. Delighted to be called upon for gran-nanny duty, I readily agreed.

At the end of February, Francis and I packed up and went to the vacation house for a few relaxing days before our babysitting stint. One day, mid-morning, I managed to skirt most of the gullies of mud on the long and hilly driveway as we set off to the market and to have lunch in Morrisville. It was a short scenic drive with lots of wide-open spaces, farmhouses and barns, but it was long enough that it felt like a little outing. A big plus of going to Morrisville would be a secluded park where Barnes could run off leash and play with other dogs. After a romp he would usually emerge smiling, his yellow coat dappled with mud.

On the way there, Francis said, "I don't feel so good."

"What's wrong, Francis?"

"Don't know. Don't feel so good."

"Is your stomach bothering you? Headache? What?" I asked.

"Don't know. Just don't feel so good."

We stopped for gas at the only station on the way to Morrisville. Francis pumped and I went inside the mini-mart to pay. The pungent smell of burnt hotdogs and sausages hung in the air. As I was bending down to the lower shelf for a Snickers bar and a Milky Way, the entrance door creaked, then slammed; a gust of wind slinked in as Francis entered. Before I could get to him, he swayed and bumped into the Marlboro cigarette case. He swayed again. His body was stiff, rigid, as he pointed one finger up towards the ceiling fan, looked up, and began turning around, around, around.

One and then two, three, four men I had not noticed came over as Francis started shaking uncontrollably, every bit of him jerking, twitching. His skin turned red. The men helped him to the floor so that he wouldn't crash onto the concrete. "Oh, my God. Oh, dear God," was all I heard myself saying around the boulder of panic lodged in my mouth. Francis was gurgling and foaming.

It seemed like a very long time before the rescue squad arrived and another long time waiting for the ambulance. The paramedics struggled with getting a blood pressure reading while I chattered nonstop, holding Francis's hand and asking, "Is he breathing? Oh, my God, is he breathing?"

I looked away from him, then swiveled back to look at him, again, again, over and over. Francis's skin became white, ghostly.

"Oh, God, oh, God, is he breathing?"

I only realized I was holding my breath when the deli lady brought me a glass of water. I had to breathe before I took a sip.

Yes, Francis was breathing. He went to the hospital in the ambulance and I followed in my car with Barnes. His CAT scan was normal. A staff doctor told me that ten percent of Alzheimer's patients have seizures and it was not likely to happen again. He added that Francis was very young for this. On the drive back to the vacation house—without groceries, without a trip to the park for Barnes, without lunch—I got some news from Francis. He told me he'd had seizures in his twenties and thirties. Then he added, "For my money, that stuff was related to drinking. I had a three, maybe four day hospital stay in upstate New York, got some medication, and that was the end of the seizures."

This sounded perfectly logical to me. I understood Francis's line of thinking. During my drinking days, I had frequently blamed any ailment or mistaken judgment on my consumption of alcohol. What he didn't tell me was that he quit those meds when the refills ran out and he couldn't use his ex-wife's prescription insurance plan. One med was for his chronic high blood pressure. The other was to prevent convulsions.

That evening Francis had trouble cutting the butternut squash. In the morning he attacked an English muffin, a Thomas's muffin, with a carving knife. I was reminded that a few days ago he came into the kitchen carrying the machete for some undetermined project.

Of course, I knew that I'd better take over use of the knives and be more attentive to dangerous situations. It made me think more about what was different with Francis. He was less attentive to me, more wrapped up in himself. He was silent so much of the time. His frustration was like a huge "No Entry" sign when he couldn't locate a word he wanted. "Can't call it up," he would say. "It's just out of reach, on the edge." I was getting reluctant to say anything that might upset him, cause him to clench his teeth and look mean, like when I suggested a shower. Sometimes his eyes were shifty. When did this stuff start? It seemed to come on overnight.

Two days after the seizure episode, we were to move in to Amy and Peter's house and be in charge of Connor and their golden retriever, Zeke; a domineering white cat, Sarah; our black cat, Philadelphia; and, as always, Barnes.

I decided that I would not mention the seizure to Peter and Amy.

We arrived the day before Peter and Amy's departure and settled in easily enough. Francis was rather quiet, which I was thankful for. If he didn't speak, he wouldn't sound confused and disoriented. I was a round-the-clock watchdog for Francis. It was okay being a watchdog for the man I loved, but it was getting tougher by the month to know what to do. Long ago, I had vowed not to be a burden to Peter; I did not discuss the demanding problems that were developing as Francis's Alzheimer's progressed.

Moments before the scheduled departure for London, Peter told me that Francis had wandered into their bedroom in the middle of the night. Peter led me outside for this conversation and I remember the bird in the nest above the back door was squawking her head off. I felt very confident that I would manage and assured Peter that we would have a wonderful time.

Of course, I could cope. I would cope.

As soon as Peter and Amy were out of sight, I loaded Connor and Francis in the car to go get ice cream. It didn't matter that it was before lunchtime, it was important to start off on the right foot.

After ice cream, Connor announced, with his three-year-old authority, that he would not be eating the yucky tuna I was preparing, or anything at all, ever. "Maybe a little more, Grammy," he said at dinner after his third portion of risotto with mushrooms.

The week was a 180-degree change of focus for me. Francis and Connor played hundreds of homemade games of hockey and golf. Hide-and-seek was always good, and Connor would have played all day long; he loved it when we got close to his hiding spot, but still didn't find him. We had snowball fights. Connor had a good arm as well as good aim, so Francis set up a target that Connor could hit and, naturally, we would miss. The snow was soft and clean, the air was crisp and not too cold. We could comfortably hike with the dogs and go sledding. I was the only one who held my breath on the slope and landed in a snow bank. When Connor napped, we all napped.

There were some difficult times, though. I tried to cover for Francis, but he could not identify his colored marker or remember the simple rules of Chutes and Ladders.

Naturally, this frustrated Connor. "Dumb. Dumb Francis. Francis doesn't listen very well. Is something wrong with your ears, Francis?"

One can't hide much from a child.

"Well, you don't listen either!" was Francis's childish retort.

For the most part, I stayed one step ahead of disruption. One rainy afternoon, though, Francis and Connor were playing checkers and suddenly checkers were flying across the living room.

Connor wailed and charged upstairs to his room.

"For heaven's sake, what happened here?" I asked.

Francis, right down at Connor's little-boy level, pouted and said, "Connor doesn't like to lose. He hit me."

Sure there was plenty of laughter, too. A cow that lived on the farm behind Peter's house wandered into the backyard. Barnes and Zeke barked furiously, spraying saliva all over the dining room windows. Connor clapped his hands and waved to the cow which stood still and stared back. That made Connor laugh even more. Soon the farmer appeared, swinging a pail of enticing cow food and they slowly sauntered off to home.

Despite trying to keep the animals confined, a fair number of times Barnes escaped to the neighbor's compost pile. My blood pressure soared when he ran across the busy road to a different, but tempting, compost pile. Being sensible cats, Sarah and Philadelphia hid somewhere upstairs for most of the week, but as soon as they ventured downstairs Barnes geared up for a frantic chase. Zeke, who lived with Sarah, slept through her quiet movements. The dogs became close buddies and snuggled up right next to each other every naptime. In the evening, one would bait the other into a playful wrestling match. Teeth were bared, grunts exploded, and fur flew in every direction until I declared biscuit-cookie-snack-time for all. The dogs knew that "biscuit" meant they should go sit by the tin of dog treats; Connor knew he should sit at the kitchen table and wait for milk and a cookie; Francis knew a snack was on the way.

The week had a nice semblance of normal living—doing what needed to be done, one day at a time—and we were all in fine fettle when Amy and Peter returned home.

A day or so after getting back to the vacation house, a noisy car announced the arrival of Lucy as it chugged up the steep, winding driveway. Lucy was a no-nonsense, cut-to-the-chase native Vermonter. She lived with her daughter and helped raise her grandchildren. She cleaned houses and was always grateful for the work she acquired. As usual, she wore holey sneakers, knee-high socks, and a bandana around her head. Lucy's voice was deep and raspy from cigarettes. Her face had wisdom lines.

In the past, Lucy and I had had discussions about who Francis was—how he fit in my life, what was happening. "Such a nice man, kind and thoughtful, and so helpful," Lucy always told me.

While Lucy was cleaning, Barnes and I headed off to the village for solitary browsing and woolgathering.

When we returned, Lucy said, "You know, he's checking out. You'd never know anything was wrong, but he hasn't got a clue. Things don't match up. I asked him if Peter had children and he told me if he had a picture he'd be able to tell how many. Then after ten or fifteen minutes, in a flash he started chuckling, smiling and telling me about Connor." She paused. "Such a nice man. What will happen?"

"We'll just take it as it comes, Lucy. One day at a time."

That afternoon, during a trip to the futon store, a salesman approached and asked, "Have you been here before?"

I said, "No."

Francis said, "Yes."

"Do you two know each other?" the salesman asked, but the humor escaped me and we left.

Damned if the same scenario didn't repeat when we arrived at the tire store.

Before we left Vermont to return to Durham, Amy and Peter

phoned and said they would come visit us in Durham for a few days in August before we all went to Emerald Isle. It was terrific news.

Friends who saw Francis regularly at A.A. meetings urged us to take a trip together while it was feasible, to take pictures, and gather up good memories to put in storage.

Of course, some acquaintances noticed Francis's increased lack of awareness and his inability to be present. He seemed to plateau at one level and then fall down to a less functioning level as he simultaneously became increasingly quiet. I compensated by talking for both of us and answering my own questions.

Our destination was Viequez, known also as the Spanish Caribbean, a gorgeous undeveloped island eight miles off the eastern coast of Puerto Rico. We flew to San Juan and from there to Viequez in an eight-seater shuttle plane over the rain forest. It felt like we could reach down and brush the mass of emerald treetops. Our taxi—and I use the word taxi very loosely—broke down five minutes after we left the tiny airport. A young, smoochie couple riding with us and returning to Viequez for the third time told us that breakdowns were ordinary. Without explanation, the driver walked off to get a brother or a cousin, a different engine, or a different car. Soon enough, he returned with a car that was in worse shape than the first but was capable of moving. We jiggled and giggled and slid our way into town on the one cow path that was called a road.

"Look how gorgeous this place is, Francis!" I said.

Flowers fell over each other everywhere, gentle shades of purples, pinks, red, orange, like a Claude Monet painting. They bloomed all along the driveway to the Inn on the Blue Horizon, which sat on an isolated perch above the serene Caribbean. The view was unobstructed for miles of multi-hued ocean that danced into a velvet blue sky. The air was clean and sweet, perfumed by the flowers. Billy Holiday played softly in the background. That night we drifted to sleep in a canopied four-poster bed dressed with elegant pastel linens, and awoke in the morning to the sounds of slapping ocean waves and whiffs of Cuban coffee. Breakfast was served by the pool—fresh strawberries, pineapples, kiwis, grapes, and avocados, accompanied by a variety of fancy eggs, breads, and meats. Heavenly.

Maggie and Charlie, the Inn's golden retrievers, figured Francis out from the get-go and, whenever we settled in by the pool, they stopped snoozing and scurried off to get a tennis ball and drop it at Francis's feet. They knew he would toss it in the pool and they would get a swim. Again. And again.

After a few false, noisy starts and stalls, I got our rented Jeep moving in a forward direction so we could jerk down the dirt road to town in search of a bakery and provisions—peanut butter, cheese, fruit, a Mountain Dew for Francis—for our picnic at the beach. Along the way we encountered island mutts and pitifully skinny cats, all scavenging. Wild ponies and big white cows with huge ears and horns meandered along the sides and into the middle of the road. It was anyone's guess what might be right around the bend.

Once Francis got out and asked a giant cow, "Would you move over?" The cow stood her ground and posed for a picture.

During the ride, I noticed Francis was counting the freckles he had since he was a kid—a habit I'd seen before—but I needed to comment anyway:

"Hey, Francis, what are ya doing?"

"Just checkin', hon. Just checkin'."

"Are you counting those spots, Francis? The dermatologist said they were fine. Freckles, Francis. Nothing to worry about. He told you to enjoy your trip to the sea. Enjoy the sun. Can you remember that? Please try to remember that."

I made an effort to hold my tongue, but it aggravated me to see Francis so intent on counting his many, many freckles, over and over again.

The bakery was opening just as we arrived. A skeletal brown and white cat slumped and sulked by the screen door. The yeasty aroma of bread hung around the tiny shop. Francis turned his attention to the large chocolate chip cookies still on the cookie sheets and asked the clerk to bag "a big one for my beautiful girl" and also one for him. The screen door banged as Francis left. When I joined him outside he was rummaging in our beach bag. "Ah ha!" he exclaimed and pulled out a well-worn long sleeve shirt—light blue, Brooks Brothers, from his days in the corporate world. He donned the old shirt over his short sleeve polo shirt and adjusted his new navy cap. "Let's go, hon. Sun's up."

It was a short and very bumpy ride to the spectacular Red Beach, which ran on forever, with sun-bleached sand that glistened like tiny fireflies and endless, mellow, aquamarine water calling out to us to come on in for a swim.

"You go on, hon. I'll sit here and watch."

"You can't be serious, Francis. Here we are, miles from home with incredible beaches to explore, on a vacation for a week in this heaven and you want to sit in a Jeep? Look. Trees for shade. Huts for our picnic lunch with the warm chocolate chip cookies. The dermatologist said you are fine. It is okay, Francis, just a little sun, Francis, and the sea you love."

I was annoyed, but he didn't appear to know it.

I slammed the door harder than I needed to, chewed on the inside of my cheek, and banged on the hood of the Jeep as I went around to open the door for Francis.

"Hi, beautiful. I love you," he said.

"Come on, Francis. Let's walk, look for shells."

He climbed out. His hand found mine. "I can swim in my shirt, and my pants, too, right, hon?'"

I didn't feel like answering his question.

We carefully positioned Francis's chair in the shade. He dozed, with his chin on his chest and his head tilted to the right. Or he gazed out at his beloved sea. Comfortable, contented to be by my side, feeling that I loved him and would keep him safe.

On our last evening, we sat in the white wooden chairs overlooking the expanse of the Caribbean, tickled by the warm and subtle evening breezes. Occasional whiffs of broiled fish and prime rib prepared by the Inn's award-winning chef came our way. Francis appeared peaceful. With my mind in neutral, I rested and relished the moment.

"Dear," Francis asked, "are we in North Carolina or South Carolina?"

It didn't bother me one little bit that he didn't know where we were. I knew where we were and I had gathered a basketful of wonderful memories.

A lesson

I lost the car.

We went to Bay, Louisiana, to visit my cousin and to housesit. It was an hour's drive into New Orleans and, after sightseeing for the day, I could not find the parking lot in the French Quarter where we had left the car. All I wanted to do was sit down on Bourbon Street and cry. This must be how Francis felt when his attempts to find something were random and repetitive, I thought. That thought made me want to cry even more.

During the same trip we met up with my college roommate, Patsy, a beautiful, honest, and straightforward person. We had not seen each other in many years but instantly fell into an easy rapport and I wanted her opinion. She said that if I hadn't told her she would not have known for sure that Francis had Alzheimer's. He seemed old and withdrawn, she noted, and he slumped and did not stand tall, as a younger person would do.

Patsy was a valuable sounding board for me as I reminisced about how he used to walk—almost strut—with a purpose. She asked me what was different now. I told her.

The more I talked, the more I realized how far away my Francis had gone. He grew upset when he couldn't buy a newspaper from a box on the street for twenty-five cents, despite the big sign that read "50¢" and he would hold his hand out, like a child, and let a shopkeeper pick out the correct amount of money when he paid for things in a store. On the airplane, he had repeatedly tried to pay for the free coffee and soft drinks, not able to remember they were free and forgetting he had no money in his pockets.

Patsy encouraged me and let me vent. I appreciated that more than she knew.

Amy, Peter, Connor, and their perpetual-motion golden retriever arrived for a visit at our house in Durham before we went to Emerald Isle for our week-long vacation.

"Come here and give me a hug, Connor." Reluctantly, he inched towards me, waved a flighty hand at Francis. "Oh, my gosh, Connor, you have grown!"

We had seen him in Vermont just a few weeks before, and it impressed me how different he looked. Maybe it was the glaring change in the relationship between Connor and Francis that I saw. Connor was demanding and petulant with Francis, who ignored him and walked away.

What bothered me even more was that Connor avoided me. I felt an uncomfortable undercurrent with Peter and Amy until we had a chance to talk. They were concerned about what they called Francis's "responsibility quotient." To Connor, Francis looked like an adult, but he didn't act like an adult, so Connor was confused and testing his boundaries. They also spoke of the difference they saw in Francis and were very worried about the situation I was in. I knew that I was trying hard to hide the changes in Francis and to deny his downward slide. Monitoring, checking on, watching, and covering for Francis more and more was not only uncomfortable for me when my family was around, but it had also become exhausting.

Early the next morning, I took the dogs for a walk and left Connor in his jammies with Francis; it had become apparent that Amy and Peter were sleeping in.

"Mom, I don't think you can leave Connor alone with Francis," Peter threw at me as soon as I returned and he caught me alone. The conversation was cut short when Connor appeared, head down, and walked over to cling to his daddy's leg.

Later, I asked Francis about the morning. "Hey, Francis, what happened when I was out with the dogs? Did you fix breakfast for Connor?"

"Sure, hon. Corn flakes. He didn't want the toast. Yucky. Burned. And he said the egg was too cold. We didn't have milk, so Connor had ice cream. He got it out."

"And I bet you had some too, Francis." I said.

"Yup, but no chocolate sauce on it."

The ice cream was really healthy low-fat frozen yogurt, but I thought it wouldn't matter to Peter so I didn't bring it up. I was certain he did not approve of Francis letting Connor take charge. We had a week ahead of us, and a peace to maintain, whatever it took.

Of course, in our beautiful falling in love days, the courtship days, Francis was charming, amusing, entertaining, always a gentleman and a delight to be with, but, I realized more and more, Peter and Amy never really knew him then.

We settled in at Emerald Isle. Francis and I had the familiar west side of the duplex and Peter and Amy had the east side. Immediately, I detected in Francis an overwhelming difference from the previous visit. This year he was cautious, slow, silent. He couldn't distinguish between the front door and the back door. I had my doubts that he had any memory of having been here before. I was now his constant point of orientation. I led. He followed. Sometimes for the hell of it I would spin around and say, "Boo!" He would laugh and stretch his arms out for a hug.

How could I help us, what could I do? Take it easy, fake it until you make it, one day at a time. Thank God for A.A. slogans and what we'd learned about powerlessness, about living and letting live, about letting go.

One time, Francis walked from the beach to the house to get the camera, but he forgot what he had gone in for. On the second trip, he couldn't find the camera. I watched Amy watching me watching Francis. And so it was.

Mid-week Francis went off by himself for a walk on the beach to get some shells. I kept looking after him. Again, Amy was watching me to see if I was watching for him. Our eyes met and I knew she understood what I was dealing with and that she would discuss it with Peter. After fifteen minutes, I decided to go find Francis. With faulty memory function, can you distinguish one beach house from another? Without a concept of time, can you judge how far you have walked? Finally, I didn't have to find him; he headed back to us.

But on other occasions he wandered off and I needed to go after him in the car. He was always delighted to see me drive up and hopped right in, just like Barnes did on the occasions when he wandered off on his own adventures. I wrote down our address and phone number and put it in Francis's pocket and hoped he would remember he had that information with him. Because wandering was a common symptom of Alzheimer's as the disease progressed, I knew Francis's wandering would likely only increase.

The surf was a decent challenge for Peter. I loved watching him ride the waves, as I had taught him to do as a toddler. At low tide, the water was warm and inviting for the rest of us to splash around in. There were movies, popcorn, s'mores, and happy, smelly dogs snoozing on the porch. Francis beat us all at miniature golf. The week, like the rambling and complicated sand castles built on the beach, disappeared quickly.

To live happily with other people one should
only ask of them what they can give.

— Tristan Bernard, L'enfant prodigue du Vesinet

Adagio/Allegro

Their days are different now:
He moves in slower pace:
She likes to run and dance,
Exulting in life's race.

Life's rhythm slows, revealing grace.
She still would run and dance,
But softly turns, to match his pace.
*Their days are different now.**

— Carmen Dressler Ward

This too shall pass

Eleven and a half months inched by, filled with:

"I'm sorry, sorry."

"It's all right, Francis."

"Where are my shoes, hon?"

"Did you leave the door open, Francis, so Barnes could take off?"

"I'm sorry."

"Please take off your wool Shetland sweater. It's warm here in North Carolina and will be over ninety degrees today. And take off that long sleeve turtleneck too, okay?"

"Why do I have to shower? No, I won't."

"Barnes wants to go for a walk now. Never mind about finding the puzzle book."

"Have to have, bring book, hon."

"Will you eat your dinner? Last time you said the spaghetti was delicious with my homemade sauce. Tomatoes and mushrooms."

"Not hungry. No. Dessert, yes."

"Where is the money I had tucked in the silver drawer for emergencies?"

"No money. What money? Money, money, money."

"Good Lord, Francis, can you hurry up so we can get to the meeting on time today?"

"Sorry. Sorry."

"Yes, yes, I love you, Francis. Plainly and simply. Yesterday and today and tomorrow. I do. I love you."

Of course, Francis used to talk and tell me what he was thinking all the time, but that changed so slowly I didn't notice. Gone were the days when we talked about everything and chatted about nothing so as to stay in sync. By spring, Francis was mostly silent. He smiled. He grinned. I started talking to him in a mothering fashion, as if he were a young boy, suggesting that he do things and telling him why. The role was frustrating for me. I eased into my day by soaking in a lilac-scented bath with a cup of coffee as early as 4:00 AM. before Francis woke up, before Barnes woke up. I wrote in my journal every morning and sometimes also at night if I still had the energy. One day at a time, I worked to keep track of and protect my Francis.

Birds began their morning trills. The dew evaporated as a spring breeze took command and made the cotton curtains sway in the guest room that doubled as an ironing room. I felt Francis standing in the doorway and staring at me. He was bundled in his white terry cloth robe and his fur-lined, squished-down-at-the-heels, L.L. Bean slippers.

"Can you show me to iron?" he asked. He often omitted or reversed the order of words in these days.

"Sure. You can work on this shirt." The shirt proved too complicated. He seemed happy when I switched him to his handkerchiefs. I retreated to the kitchen, and turned on the radio for company while I made my never-the-same-but-always-good meatloaf. The hamburger and eggs were out of the refrigerator and I was looking for breadcrumbs when it felt too quiet.

"Francis? Francis, where are you?" I called out, but knew he was gone. I took the stairs two at a time, turned off the iron, glimpsed his bathrobe hung in the closet, and saw that his khakis and yesterday's shirt were gone from the chair.

"Come on, Barnes, let's go find Francis." We drove around and around again in the neighborhood. No Francis. I chewed a piece of gum. Double Bubble. Another piece. Blew bubbles. Drove. Went home. Called the police. Went out. Searched again. Asked people, asked children, "Where is Francis?" We were new in the neighborhood. Did anyone even know Francis? Nobody knew about his Alzheimer's except our neighbors next door and they were away.

Back home to check phone messages. Discovered Francis's medical alert bracelet with his name, address, and phone number on his bureau. Four hours vanished. I set out again. Then, oh, my God, thank you, God, I spotted him standing stone still at the curb of a four-lane street. Would he walk into the traffic? I held my breath, drove up to him, swung open the passenger door.

Francis smiled, slid in, and reached for the seat belt. "How've you been, hon? Pretty day," he said.

"Where were you going, Francis? Did you know you were leaving? It scared me, frightened me. Tell me, Francis, please. What can we do?"

"Well, we'll have to…"

I remembered his exact words, his pause, and then there were no words as tears dribbled down his cheek and he dug in his pocket for a handkerchief.

Francis was quiet, at sixes and sevens it seemed, prior to the arrival of his middle daughter, Carolyn, her husband, Jack, and their fourteen-month-old daughter, Debra. He mowed half of the lawn and swept half of the deck, while I prepared salads for luncheon and set the table.

Carolyn had a big, beautiful smile on her face as she hopped out of their car, and I liked her instantly. As soon as there was an opportunity, Jack commented to me about how quiet Francis had become and I explained that Francis's silence had notably increased since Christmas. Carolyn commented that her Dad sometimes responded twenty minutes after she had asked him a question. It was comfortable talking to them. I sensed they cared about Francis.

Grandbaby Debra stole the show. She perched in her Pops' arms and giggled and flirted with him as he blew air kisses to her. She exuded delight when he held her tight and she squinched up her shoulders, touched his lips, and poked his cheeks with her chubby fingers. Pops glowed.

During lunch, Debra was in a highchair when Barnes came over to lick her wiggly, bare toes. Wordlessly, Francis got up from his chair and put Barnes out into the back yard. I guessed that although Francis could not easily communicate verbally, he had clear thoughts that Barnes was bothering his granddaughter so he took action. After dessert we went to the playground so Debra could go on the swing. Francis and Jack tossed tennis balls for Barnes until he wallowed and rolled like a pig in a five-inch deep mud puddle he managed to uncover. Then we took Barnes swimming.

Carolyn nodded me toward a private place and said, "Only once in a while do I recognize my Dad. He follows you everywhere, like a puppy dog. What's to come?" I emphasized that we needed to focus on staying in the present and keeping Francis from getting too frustrated, and I promised to give her *The Thirty-Six Hour Day*, the bible for Alzheimer's caregivers.

It was a sad and poignant moment for me when Carolyn, Jack, and Francis were sitting on the lawn—the mowed part—playing with Debra. I came out of the house to take Barnes for a walk. I expected Francis to stay and visit more with his family, but he got up and chose to walk with me, as Carolyn had said, like a puppy dog.

After the hugs and goodbyes, Carolyn said, "You'll have to come to Denver." Those were the sweetest words I could have heard.

Before bed, we talked about the visit. I asked about the day. Francis commented on this and that and after a while he told me Carolyn had come to visit.

"Who else was here, Francis?"

"Jack." A vague look crossed Francis's face before he added, "I can't say about that crowd." That was my signal that Francis could not give me additional details or tell me about his granddaughter, Debra. Our conversation was over.

Of course, never did I think that Francis was withholding information or that he chose to ignore my inquiry. Somehow, I could tell that he gave me all he knew.

If Carolyn had come the previous summer, as had been the original plan, she would have seen a different man. He had been carefree, happy. He had dismissed from his mind problems he recognized but could not solve. By the time she did visit, Francis's world had become blander. Simple living skills were a big challenge. He did not seem to understand or pay attention to what I said, so I repeated things, slowly and distinctly, as if I were speaking to a foreigner who needed time to translate. There were times when I preferred being silent rather than suffer through his halted and incomplete responses.

Of course, Francis continued to change. Gradual changes I didn't see or wouldn't look at. Did Francis know he was behaving differently? If he did, he wasn't telling. We were building a silent cocoon.

And of course, I felt alone, alone with only the physical being of Francis and grateful for the unending attention from Barnes and his chunky, otter-like slapping tail.

My second grandchild was due to be born in early June and I had agreed to be a gran-nanny helper and stay with the family for his arrival. I researched assisted-living facilities close to Burlington, Vermont, and found The Pillars with its lovely bucolic grounds just south of town in Shelburne. It was unsecured; residents stayed there voluntarily. I said to Francis, "We are going to Vermont in a few weeks for the arrival of Amy and Peter's new baby and I have found a great place for you to stay for a couple of days while I help out. It's like a bed and breakfast and the grounds are lovely. They will fix your meals and see that you get your meds on schedule. We can talk on the phone whenever you wish, then I'll pick you up in a couple of days and we'll go to the vacation house for a few days, okay?"

I thought—hoped—Francis said "Okay," but maybe he just said "Oh." I reviewed the plan with him a number of times before we left Durham and began the nine hundred mile drive to Vermont.

Two days before we were to go to The Pillars, availability there was postponed, so we spent an extra weekend in the vacation house. I was on pins and needles, anticipating how things would work out with The Pillars as well as waiting for news about the arrival of the baby.

I phoned Connor and invited him to go to Pizza Putt.

"Francis won't be there, just you and me?" Connor queried.

"Yes, Connor. Just you and me."

"All right, Grammy! When can we go?"

"Now, Connor. Now."

I hoped Francis would be safe enough in the vacation house with the television tuned to his favorite channel and bagels on the kitchen counter. The cat stayed with him. Barnes rode shotgun with me and listened patiently as I reminded him how important he was to me and how I appreciated his thumping tail and his unexpected sloppy kisses. I reminded him that he should stop teasing the cat. I was buoyed up by the crisp air, the sunlight, the prospect of a fun afternoon with my grandson. I felt free.

Every time he beat me at a hole of miniature golf, Connor got kiddy-giddy and jumped up and down, and wiggled a loosy-goosy dance. The ordinary pizza was enhanced by happy, noisy kids. At his house, Connor raced in to tell his parents how he beat me on ALL the holes of golf.

"Hi, Francis. I'm home."

"Oh, where ya been?" he asked without getting up off the sofa, in contrast to the days when he hurried to me and welcomed me with a big hug and a kiss.

Later, I set about packing for our trip home. My final goodbye to the Jeffersonville house was near at hand. It would be Don's as part of our divorce settlement. Many memories had been made in that house: soaking in the hot tub, sculpting buxom snow ladies on the deck when Francis and I were blessed with enough snow, staring into the sparkling, moon-lit sky, struggling with the nearly impass-able hilly driveway covered in ice, vacationing with friends in sum-mers, vacationing alone with Barnes—my anchor throughout it all.

I was lolling in the Jacuzzi, one of my favorite activities, the loud jets masking all other sound, so Francis took the call from Peter. Samuel Mathew Young, a handsome, healthy 8 pound and 6 ounce, 21 inch baby greeted the world at 4:43 AM. It was June 11, 1998.

The time had come to spring into action and go to The Pillars. During the drive, I clutched the steering wheel while jabbering with nervousness and singing along with the radio. I didn't want to give Francis any opportunity to say he wouldn't stay there. At least he had willingly packed a small overnight case and put it in the car.

In the admissions office, as I was filling out the paperwork, out of the corner of my eye I noticed Francis shaking his head.

"Not staying," he mouthed and then announced it. His arm was like cement when I touched him.

"Francis, you know you need someone to prepare your meals and to set out your meds for you. I will only be gone a couple of days," I explained. "Amy and Peter are counting on me to help with the new baby and I promised I would be there. Please understand why I am asking you to stay here. It's just for a couple of nights. I love you and I need someone to care for you for just a short time. Please, Francis. It's a beautiful place here. Please."

A mask of fear veiled his face, a look I had never seen before. I recalled that at an Alzheimer's Management Convention we had been advised to never argue with a patient. I solicited The Pillars personnel for help and was reminded they could only keep him if he agreed to stay. Francis glared at me and accused me of springing this on him. Round and round we went. I was livid that he would not, could not, comply. Never had I seen Francis like this, ready to explode. Without a word, he picked up his suitcase and headed out the door toward the car. The staff called his behavior "eloping."

Of course, I was not pleased that my connection with Francis was interfering with my ability and desire to carry out my commitment and be available to Amy and Peter and Connor when my new grandbaby arrived. Maintaining a close and strong relationship with my family was of utmost importance to me and I was very frustrated with the situation I was in. Why the hell couldn't Francis stay at the Pillars just for one night? What did it mean to him that I didn't see?

We chatted beside my Volvo with a pleasant resident whom I suspected the staff had sent out to try to persuade Francis to stay. He said, "Hello, my name is Ernest and I hope you will stay with us for a few days. I've been here a couple of years and it's good. They have bus trips into Burlington whenever you want to go. The food is good, very good. There's a nice bunch of guys I've become friends with. Come on, I'll show you around."

Francis was cordial. He put his suitcase in the car and then agreed to stay for lunch. Just lunch. I had from noon to three with my new grandson. The staff had shown Francis a room while he was there, but he was adamant about leaving and being with me. It didn't occur to me to simply not return at the agreed upon time, just to be late.

That evening, I tersely asked Francis how his day went.

"A nice day, wasn't it? There was a lunch, hon."

Never before had I been so furious at Francis. He didn't have a clue what was bothering me. It only made it worse to know that he couldn't help it. Powerlessness is what we are supposed to learn in A.A., but this was beyond my ability to accept and I was at a top level of angry. While aggressively chewing a piece of gum, I missed and chomped a bloody gash on the side of my tongue.

Francis looked angelic as he easily fell asleep. I repeated the serenity prayer for as long as I could, mumbling it in my head before I drifted in and out of a restless doze until dawn.

To make it easier to visit my family frequently and stay as long as I wanted without disrupting their household, I bought a condo. The location was perfect, less than fifteen minutes from Peter's house and downtown Burlington, and just a few steps into Red Rocks Park, with its trees and trails and access to Lake Champlain, a dog heaven. My condo was high on a hill with views over rooftops. I could pretend to jump from my deck onto a floating cloud to play in the sky.

With Francis as a helper, moving in was one giant challenge after another. Furniture from my marital home that had been in storage was delivered to the condo's garage. Francis was great about hauling the furniture around, but the second he was out of my sight he relocated the cartons I had put in the kitchen or the bedroom and denied touching them. Frequently, they ended up in the basement or back in the garage. One morning, I raised my voice at him. He shot me a menacing look, stomped off, and headed down the hill out of the condo complex. Most of the time, Francis was easygoing and cheerful, but a different personality was making more and more of an appearance.

"Maybe we should get a bell to put on Francis so we would know when he's leaving us," I said jokingly to Barnes as we prepared to go hunt for Francis. Although he had walked with us in Red Rocks Park, it seemed unlikely that being a city boy, he would venture into the woods alone. I called the Burlington police. Was it being uncaring or simply reasonable when I decided not to drive after him and search around the adjoining neighborhoods as I had done a couple of times at home in North Carolina?

"Here he is, miss. I found this very nice young gentleman down in the supermarket inspecting the corn. Glad to be of service," the policeman said. Francis stood by silently.

"Where'd you go, Francis?" I asked.

"Oh, to the senior center. And I watched the boats on the lake. Missed you." Francis said this matter-of-factly. He beamed his I-adore-you smile and that made me smile, too. But the senior center was in North Carolina and we were in Vermont. Lake Champlain was close enough to the condo, but I didn't believe he could have found it by himself.

Wandering was a common symptom; I had been forewarned. Apparently a new phase had arrived, in that Francis acted as if it were fine, even normal, for him to take off, to "elope." He'd taken a bigger step down the path to nowhere. It had been depressing at the Alzheimer support meetings to be regaled with the devastating behaviors that could be expected. A.A. suggested living one day at a time, and that was the plan I tried to adopt for us.

I wanted to at least accomplish some minimal organization at the condo before we headed back to Durham, but Francis demanded more and more of my attention. The Red Cross ran a voluntary day care program in Colchester, north of Burlington, for people who needed supervision. Francis agreed to give it a try for a few days. Many of the participants enrolled in the program were severely handicapped, physically and mentally. Francis appeared to be very much out of place. He was polite and sociable and acted normal to the unobservant eye. Towards the end of the week a staff nurse called me and reported that Francis was irritable, pacing, too agitated to participate in their program, and eloping whenever he saw a chance, refusing to return to the center. For my peace of mind, she suggested I should call his doctor and get some medications to calm him. His doctor was in North Carolina. We needed to go home.

Of course, I knew what had to be done eventually and eventually was fast approaching. I promised Amy and Peter that I would look for an assisted-living community as soon as we returned to Durham. I was tired, so very tired of trying to take care of us, but thoughts of assisted living made me feel like sobbing. It used to be that I could look at Francis, at a party, on a bus, by the sea, and know what he was thinking. "How come you can always get into my head?" he frequently said. How could I care for him if I didn't know what he was thinking and he couldn't tell me? Additionally, he had gotten slow, so slow. Some days he stood in front of his closet for a long time before he decided what to wear and then changed pants two or three times within the hour. Or he opened and closed the same kitchen cupboards looking for a coffee cup. I sensed his confusion as his posture stiffened, but I didn't know when I should step in and take over the task . When I was overtired I got annoyed more easily and forgot how devastating his loss of abilities must feel.

Francis's mood in general seemed to improve when we were on more familiar turf at home. One hot and especially humid Saturday morning, Francis was puttering around outside, sweeping the porch and the driveway. Suddenly, he hurried in and went straight upstairs. I finished the kitchen chores in about ten minutes then found him flopped spread eagle on our bed, ghostlike, ashen, still.

"Francis? Francis, how are you?"

"I don't, I don't know."

Frantic, I phoned 911. Francis did not respond any further than saying, "That's my love, Mary Ann," when the rescue squad questioned him and took him to the ER in Chapel Hill.

"Quick, quick, Barnes, come with me to the hospital. Ride shotgun, Barnes, I'm so scared, so scared." It helped to put my hand on Barnes's head.

Was it heat exhaustion? A small stroke? No one was able to determine what had happened and Francis had zero recollection of any part of the day. "Watch him," I was advised.

"Francis, I think this is a sign you need more care than I can give you," I whispered.

"I think so," he said as tears trickled across his pale cheeks.

Of course, I whispered. I didn't want to say it. I didn't want my Francis to hear it.

At first we went everywhere together, within 150-mile radius of our home, in search of an assisted-living facility with an Alzheimer's wing that accepted Medicare. This was a tough job. It was somewhat easier for me to have Francis along because I concentrated on his reactions, and pretended it was just another outing, an event that killed time, and ended with lunch or a visit to TCBY for cones. The charade didn't work for long. Most of the facilities we visited were not acceptable as a place to visit briefly, let alone for an extended and undetermined amount of time. I could not tap into Francis's thoughts, but my thoughts were horrible enough. How would it ever be possible to leave him in one of the places we had seen? It became too difficult for either one of us to voice our opinions or even speak at all. After these inspections, we slouched on the concrete bench outside TCBY and silently stared at each other as our frozen yogurt cones melted and Barnes worked at licking up the drips off the sidewalk. Eventually, I took on the depressing task with just Barnes for company. I never made an appointment, preferring to drop in to get a gut reaction about the daily ambiance. I always visited the ladies room and the dining area to check for general cleanliness.

My hopes were over-the-top high that an interview with social services would lead us to an acceptable assisted-living facility. When we arrived at the office, the sky was overcast and rain was in the forecast. The building looked more dismal than at our previous visit two years ago.

"Have a seat," the receptionist said. I scanned the crowded room and we settled in for a long wait. A couple of hours later, a side door opened, a worker stuck her head out and bellowed, "Tomson, Frank Tomson." Now was the hour.

Miss Smith, a social worker, sat behind a neat and too tidy desk. She was prim in her beige suit. A floral scarf brightened her outfit and her smile was warm and friendly. I was willing to bet she was fairly new at the job, but I didn't ask. A scraggly bunch of fake fall flowers sat on the sill in front of a dirty window. Beige defined the office, the walls, the chairs, the floor, all beige. Lacking hope.

The application process began with questions directed to Frank.

"Your name and date of birth?"

"Well, I'm about fifty...and a half."

"You're sixty-three, Francis," I interjected.

"Single, married, widowed, or divorced?"

"Widowed."

"You're divorced, Francis."

"Date of divorce?"

"I'll have to get that for you," I said and added that since Francis had applied for disability two years ago this information must be in his file.

"Oh, well, this is the way we do it," Miss Smith informed us and the questions continued. Then Miss Smith explained the process: "Now this application will go to Raleigh for approval but you don't have much time to find a place for him. The approval is only good for thirty days."

"What if I can't find a suitable place in thirty days?" I asked.

"You just come back when your paperwork expires and we start again."

Miss Smith smiled.

The next day I started telephoning every assisted-living facility listed in the telephone book. Added to my criteria of an Alzheimer's wing and acceptance of Medicare was the availability of Medicaid beds since Francis did not have the funds for a private pay facility. When I got affirmative replies, I set out to visit. Sometimes I didn't bother to go in. Sometimes I left after I opened the front door and got a whiff of the corridor or visited the rest room. There were a few vague promises of expected vacancies.

I phoned Miss Smith to express my dismay and learned that Francis's social security benefit of $800 per month was too high for him to qualify for the Medicaid bed I had been trying to find for him. In addition, she informed me that Medicaid beds are usually given to patients who are already in the facility. "The only way you get a bed for Mr. Tomson is if he is hospitalized for three days. Then the hospital is responsible for placing him."

I laughed and said, "Hospitalization, Miss Smith, is not likely. What other options do I have?"

"Or you have him declared incompetent, a ward of the state, and the state finds him a placement."

No bloody way would I even think of such an action.

"Then there's private pay, starting at about $3,000 per month base fee."

Miss Smith had just heard about a facility in Marion, in the farthest northwest corner of North Carolina. It was private pay, but cheaper, and it might be suitable, at least for short term. We should visit. "Don't forget that Mr. Tomson will need to have a physical exam, a tuberculosis test, other tests, and a number of government forms signed by a doctor within thirty days of admission to any facility," Miss Smith added.

Armed with a cooler filled with pretzels, energy bars, Good &

Plentys, Milk Bones for Barnes, and Mountain Dew for Francis, we left home at daybreak on a Sunday morning to visit the facility in Marion. I reasoned that it was cheaper because of its remote location. My expectations were high as I envisioned a quaint, bucolic town, and a welcoming bed-and-breakfast type facility. My mother's name was Marion with an O. As if that would help. It never occurred to me to check the traffic report, but the drive was annoyingly arduous, with lines of cars at a standstill because of long stretches of road repair. Barnes was content, curled up on his blanket in the back seat and Francis had a crossword puzzle book—a beginner one—on his lap, a book we could work on together. I tried to think positive thoughts and just drive. Drive.

To break up the monotonous trip, we stopped to let Barnes get out and to buy peaches at a roadside stand and to chat with the farmer about how to store them so they would not spoil as fast. He told us to put them on a plate and not have them touch. I suggested we take some to the receptionist at our destination.

My hopes plummeted and I slowed the car as we approached the outskirts of the dilapidated and deserted town of Marion and found the tall red brick hospital building. The grounds were clean but barren. A weary looking woman, wearing a tattered apron over her calico housedress, sat on the porch in one of six green plastic chairs. A solitary pale pink geranium slumped in a grungy pot.

"Hello," Francis said.

"Hey," I said.

No reply.

The front door was loose on its hinges. We entered, rang the bell for the receptionist.

"Why, now, thanks to you for them peaches and I'll take you to third floor. I'll get the key for the elevator. We got the Alzheimer's up there. Up on three."

We followed the receptionist around the corner to the elevator and stared as she unlocked and tugged on the door to open it, and then struggled to close it. When we were encased within, I reached for Francis's hand and he gave me a squeeze as we rumbled and jerked upward. Slowly. I wanted to go back downstairs, fast, out the door, leave, dismiss Marion. I acted calm for Francis's sake, but I don't think I fooled him at all.

A group of people who looked like derelicts stared at us when we arrived in the Alzheimer's unit. We rounded a corner and came upon four women sprawled on a wooden bench and another woman bent over so far in her wheelchair that her spiky brown hair almost brushed the floor. "Sit up, Mary," the one visible nurse admonished.

"Here's the eating area. We have two feedings. They usually sweep up after the feedings," our somewhat embarrassed guide told us as Francis and I gawked at the dirty dishes and remnants of past "feedings" on the tables and the floor.

Silently, we followed the guide down the dingy hall. It was impossible to ignore the diapers rolled up and stashed on windowsills, unmade beds with dirty linens, the stink in the air.

"The activities director is off on Sundays. I guess we have an empty bed. It's private pay at $1,350 per month. Meds, incidentals are extra, laundry, too. Do you wanna see the laundry? The kitchen's locked now. You can visit here anytime, you know, anytime."

I declined a visit to the laundry. It had been a mistake to assume the fee was lower than other private institutions because of the location. Francis contributed a too-loud "Bye-bye."

Barnes stuck his nose out the window as we approached the car, then leaned over the seat and gave us both sloppy kisses.

Squeaky windshield wipers punctuated the black silence on our three-hour ride home.

Francis arranged and rearranged the peaches, then did it again, as I prepared supper.

One day at a time

Southern House was a chain of private-pay assisted-living residences that fell in the category of rest homes and did not qualify for Medicaid. However, they had separate Alzheimer's units, dubbed the Discovery Rooms. I learned of a vacancy in the newer Southern House, fifty-eight miles south of our home in Durham and, with Barnes riding shotgun, I hurried off to inspect it. It was a Godsend. The grounds were attractive and I sighed audibly when I entered the lobby, smelled the fresh bouquet of flowers on a pretty cherry table, and caught strains of Mozart. On my right was a richly paneled library with plenty of books, a small television, comfortable wing chairs by the fireplace, and a board game, without players, set up on a card table. The wallpaper was tasteful; geometric designs in a restful blue. Bright and cheerful pottery bowls filled with potpourri were in the A-plus bathroom. The Southern House was designed to resemble a fine bed and breakfast and it succeeded. It was reminiscent of the numerous bed and breakfasts we visited in our early courting days. Surely this facility would appeal to my Francis. But where were the people?

The admissions director, Pam, welcomed me cheerfully. She was dressed in a navy blue, tailored suit, and wore sensible shoes. Her long, fashionably blond hair was tied back with a red and yellow striped scarf. I guessed she was in her late twenties. Her self-confidence was evident, and she had the aura and enthusiasm that went along with being successful at her job. We discussed Francis and she proposed that initially he could go in the general independent living section, which would give him freedom to go in and out and around the facility whenever he pleased. If that didn't work, he could easily be moved to the secured Discovery Room, the Alzheimer's unit.

Pam took me on a tour. The dining room could have been part of any home-style restaurant. There were tables for four or six, small vases of flowers as centerpieces. At noon, it was filled with recently coiffed grey-haired ladies, who wore their pearls and skirt-and-sweater sets, and men in tailored pants, shirts with open collars under old-man cardigan sweaters, buttoned half way up. The air was filled with the aroma of just-baked chocolate chip cookies.

The Alzheimer's unit—the Discovery Room—was circular, a thoughtful consideration so that patients could walk, or pace, without bumping into walls or getting stuck in dead-end corridors. The large common room had hallways off of it leading to the semi-private bedrooms and an inviting outdoor patio and garden area with flowers and another circular walkway.

The Alzheimer's patients there were presentable, though a bit hodgepodge. Maybe their socks didn't match, but I didn't see anyone angry or crying in a corner. They had gathered close to a long table with sandwich preparations for lunch. I felt like an intruder, invading the residents' privacy. I tried not to gape. I wanted to be polite, to linger, to make eye contact, but I was uncomfortable. There was a kitten to focus on, and I did so while I chattered to Pam and heard only my own voice. I wanted to believe Francis belonged here. I wanted to let loose and sob, to run back into our carefree courting days.

Of course, I noticed that the exterior looked good. But, my God, what a horrible way to spend the last of one's days, living with a group of strangers who have an enormous variety of ever-changing quirky issues, being locked in an area with no way out unless someone accompanies you, probably just for a miserable doctor's appointment. It consoled me that possibly the disease let its captive ignore and forget the lousy stuff and just stay in a present moment, waiting for the next chocolate chip cookie.

An interview for Francis was scheduled for the end of the week. Much too frequently, I nervously explained to Francis that this was a temporary arrangement while I went to New Jersey to finalize my divorce. At a minimum of $3,000 per month, we could not afford it for long.

As I hoped he would, at first glance Francis wholeheartedly approved of the appearance of Southern House. He impressed Pam with his gentlemanly manner and appropriate comments. Abruptly he sat up straighter. He began asking Pam personal questions. Francis's voice grew stronger and I realized that he had fallen into his former role as an executive search recruiter and Pam was his candidate. Pam looked at me with a what's-going-on-here expression on her face. I shrugged and steered the discussion toward choosing a date for moving in. We left swiftly, a smidgen shy of being rude.

"Come on, Francis. Let's go to bed." I stopped myself before reminding him that early in the morning we would go to Southern House. "Will you help me get our frozen yogurt?" It was 7:00 PM. He used to serve me frozen yogurt in a cereal bowl, two giant scoops with a generous blob of Dream Whip, decorated with both rainbow and chocolate sprinkles. Then he'd call upstairs and ask if I wanted hot fudge or butterscotch sauce. Sometimes he would put a rosebud or a chocolate chip cookie on the tray. Always he delivered it with a smile and a smooch. These evenings, I pried the lid off the frozen yogurt container for him, guided his hand on the ice cream scoop, watched as he chased chocolate chunks or caramel ripples with a spoon, and popped the booty into his mouth.

Take it easy

On the day of Francis's relocation, August 10, 1998, I started in on the general morning chores, feeling more numb and empty than I could have ever imagined. His bag was packed and in the car. I knew the challenge had just begun. Flashes of the fiasco at The Pillars burst into my head repeatedly. Francis's compliance with the plan to stay at the Southern House surprised me until I realized he probably didn't grasp the meaning of it. As for me, I was caught in the mode of doing what had to be done. I was so wrapped up in how I was going to get Francis settled, worried about whether the independent living section would work for him, that I did not—could not—think about what was happening to us for the long ride.

"Today is the day we go to Southern House, Francis," I said.

"Yes, my love, I know," he replied, but I didn't know if packing his suitcase meant anything more to him than just a job, a task without meaning. Did he understand that Southern House was assisted living for him? Or was it just a big bed and breakfast, like the many we had visited? I dared not speak of it more. I feared what he might say. He had gotten very silent, but that didn't mean he wasn't thinking. Or did it?

As Francis was dressing, I retreated outside to the deck. It was a private space, surrounded by overgrown forsythia, the graceful branches dancing in the breeze. Birds chirped, seemed to answer each other. I stretched, closed my eyes, basked in the warmth of the early morning August sun. I was wearing my pink floral shortie nightgown and the matching flimsy silk robe, an outfit I bought to be coquettish when Francis invited me to accompany him on a business trip to Philadelphia, six or maybe eight years ago. During the timeless years. When we were simply falling in love and living one day at a time.

My coffee grew tepid. On an ordinary day, Francis would fill my cup when he returned from sweeping the driveway. And he was always sweeping, forever sweeping. Soothingly sweeping. Ours was, hands down, the cleanest driveway in the neighborhood, maybe in the whole town. In the beginning days, Francis swept with a bounce in his step, like he was dancing with the broom. This morning, he jabbed and jerked the broom across the driveway, pushed the bristles, pulled the bristles, pushed, pulled, swished. He practically attacked the driveway. I knew he was sweeping it for the last time. Did Francis know? Where was his ordinary, if sparse, chatter? I guessed he sensed that something was not right about this day but couldn't fill in the blank space.

On an ordinary day, Francis would lean the broom against the garage, take off his white denim hat, and shove it in the back pocket of his khaki shorts. He'd push back some stray hairs, find me, and ask about a snack or breakfast or lunch or a ride in the car to nowhere in particular.

Barnes was restless, no doubt sensing my mood and that something was out of the ordinary. His head rested on my foot, but he was ready to jump into go mode as soon as I gave the slightest clue. I wanted to get on with the ugly things on the day's agenda.

Pam greeted us in the driveway at the Southern House, and immediately whispered to me that she wanted some reassurance from me that Francis would stay willingly and not wander off. She could not begin to imagine how fervently I hoped that he would be able to manage independent assisted living.

The second we were alone in Francis's private room, he put his arms out and came to me, with his unforgettable let's-make-love look. I ducked away and chattered about the comfortable room, the private bathroom, the shower, and even the freshly painted walls. "Oh, dear, dear, where is your bureau? Gosh, how can I unpack your duffle, Francis, where will I put things? I'll bring pictures. Which ones would you like, do you think?" I rambled on and on as he shadowed me with outstretched arms, ready for an embrace. Then I was alone.

Francis had gone into the hall and was headed toward an exit sign, not running, but walking at a fast clip. I followed, out the door, around the back of Southern House. I called to him. He turned and looked at me but kept going, faster, through the shrubs in the gardens, and past the front entry and the windows of the admissions office.

"Will you stay here, Francis?" I asked when I caught up to him.

"I don't know that."

Pam appeared.

"I think we need the Discovery Room," she said.

A repeating image of Francis crowded my mind: I saw him wheeling his meager belongings piled helter-skelter on a noisy cart, away from the independent living bedroom, past the upscale independent living dining room, and headed for his lunch, lunch behind a locked door. I saw a grown man, then I blinked and saw him as a three-year-old, in little boy denim shorts, a Lone Ranger T-shirt, and cowboy boots, steering a red wheelbarrow on a playground. What if he said no? What if he sat down, slammed his heels into the floor, and wailed that he wouldn't stay?

"Thank you, no, I won't be staying for lunch, no, but thanks, yes, thanks, Pam, for the invitation, Pam, " I stammered.

The speedometer tickled eighty miles per hour as I raced away to my home.

Five o'clock that evening a phone call came from the staff at Southern House.

"We want you to know that Mr. Frank is fine. He had two suppers, two, bussed the tables, rubbed a lady's cold hand. He makes people smile."

Of course, I was glad to hear that Francis was fine. I wasn't fine. I didn't want to have supper alone. My whole body felt cold, shivery. I grew up in a real house, a house with substance, character, and family in Bridgeport, Connecticut. This little dwelling in Durham was okay with Francis in it, but now it felt hollow. For the past eighteen months, my focus had been Francis. Even when he couldn't tell me what he'd been doing or what he wanted, at least he was here. A body, somewhat pudgy and balding, but until very recently he welcomed me with open arms, a smile. Now what?

The night was long and fretful. I nestled into Francis's side of the bed, tossed, turned.

Night passed. Morning arrived.

The phone rang. Seven o'clock and it was another call from Southern House. One of the staff reported that Frank had given them a real scare, that he had had "one of his fits" and was on the way to the hospital.

"He seemed good by the time he left here but we wanted you to know." The staff person spoke as if fits were a common thing with Francis.

Barnes and I hurried off to the emergency room at the hospital near Southern House. The doctor told me that Francis' blood tests indicated that his Dilantin, the medication to prevent seizures, was too low and he asked whether Frank had missed last night's dosage. "Frank has to have a local doctor," the hospital doctor added. "We can give you a referral, but most offices around here are full and won't take any new patients. Sorry to tell you this, but that's the way it is around here." I could not believe what he said. Again we needed a solution.

When I got to Francis, he was standing up and pulling at the IV tube, ready to leave the hospital. Unshaven and in rumpled clothes, he looked like Nicholas Cage as a convict on the run, but after he was cleared to leave the hospital, I took him to lunch anyway, to a Southern Chicken and Barbeque Hut. To make conversation, I asked about how his night had been, what he had for dinner, what the other residents were like. In lieu of any answers, he gave me a vacant smile. He ate his lunch with gusto and struggled to get the Sarah Lee pecan pie out of its container. "Good idea, my love," he said when I suggested he eat it right from its little package.

What a long way we had come, I thought, as I pictured the white linen tablecloths, the professional waiters with black bow ties in the upscale Luger Steak House in Manhattan, the slabs of beef we picked out before they grilled it, the creamy spinach, Francis's favorite hash browned potatoes. Was there dessert? Always.

We returned to the Discovery Room. I kept my arm around Francis while I discussed his medications with the staff. My mind raced. Who was supervising his care? Why was his Dilantin level low? Where could I find a local doctor?

"I'll call you soon, Francis," I said, gave him a kiss and turned to leave.

"How will I get home?" he said.

I managed to get an appointment for the following week with a nurse practitioner at a clinic in McGee Corners, close to the Southern House. Before we got there, Francis had another seizure and was back in the emergency room. Meanwhile, I called Dr. Eveymore in Durham to discuss what was happening. He didn't think Frank was having seizures and he said he would call Southern House and adjust the Dilantin medication. Thankfully, he agreed to cover Francis until I could find a local physician.

A phone call from my Francis: "I love you so, I miss you so. Whew. This place!" he said. "I'll tell you all about it when I get home." His expectation about returning home, which I knew could not happen, saddened me as I acknowledged that I was no longer able to keep us safe, as I had promised two years ago when we had discussed our future.

Within a day or two another phone call from Southern House: "Mr. Frank had a fainting spell. He's better now and wants to talk to you." Was the fainting spell the same as what a different aide called a fit?

"Hi, love. I'm not so good. Can you come down here?"

"Certainly, Francis, soon. Can you watch the golf tournament for a while?"

Soon another call: Francis was at the hospital again. By now, I knew the route to the hospital without paying much attention to where I was going. Again, his Dilantin level was much lower than the therapeutic level.

In a couple of days, we were at the McGee Corners Clinic, on the wrong day. My anxiety had played tricks on me. We sat and fidgeted all afternoon waiting to be squeezed in for a very short visit with a nurse practitioner. She increased the Dilantin dosage.

At a follow up visit the next week as soon as we sat down in the office, Francis asked for some razor blades.

Good God, is he suicidal? I thought.

He reached into his pocket, pulled out his razor and explained that he couldn't find his Dopp kit and he wanted to shave.

The nurse practitioner skirted the blades request, checked his

Dilantin level, increased the dosage, and was alarmed by his high blood pressure. Dr. Eveymore had felt Francis's chronic high blood pressure should be left alone, and I persuaded the nurse practitioner to just make one change at a time. We left and went into the tiny town of Springfield to get a haircut for Francis. My Francis, my dapper Francis had always cared about his appearance.

"Hey, good looking," I called to him when I returned to the barber shop. "Are you game for an ice cream cone? Chocolate?" And behold! A sparkle in his eyes, a sweet small smile, and an affirmative nod.

When I next visited Francis at the Discovery Room, I was struck with the impression that he had shrunk. Could that possibly happen in a few days or had I not noticed it before? He hardly hugged me back as I embraced him.

Of course I wondered, I worried. What the hell was happening? What could I do?

On the day of the next appointment with the nurse practitioner, Francis took cautious baby steps, tucked his chin into his neck, and swayed. My arm was tight around him as we inched towards my car. As soon as we got the seatbelt secured, his body sagged and he drooped like a sunflower in need of a healthy drink of water. At the appointment, the nurse practitioner was pleased that his blood pressure had improved and left his Dilantin as it was prescribed.

I had to hold on and guide Francis as he shuffled back towards the Discovery Room. I blew him a bunch of kisses, told him I would be back very soon, and hurried away. For a moment, I glimpsed the first air kiss he had blown to me in the taxicab the day he told me, plainly and simply, that he was in love with me.

A black and giant shadow arrived and circled over my head. Clearly Francis would not be able to go to Emerald Isle with me, Barnes, and our friends Helen and Jack, as was planned for next week. Most importantly, I had the challenge of finding a Medicaid bed for my love in a suitable long-term facility.

Despite the fact that Francis had minimal contact with his three adult children, I felt obliged to notify them of the situation. Communication had been easy with Carolyn when she brought her family to visit her dad, so I phoned her. She offered to help financially, but their budget was already tight. I went on to explain that her Dad would need to be in a long-term care facility and asked if one of the children would want him located close to them. Carolyn said she would talk to Ronald and Claudia. Within a couple of days, Carolyn reported back that they were not interested in helping financially. In regard to having their father near by, the answers were no, no, and no.

Of course I threw the ball to Francis's children to see what they would do. Honestly, I knew I would not let him move out of my sight. Nor would he move out of my heart.

I had made a reservation to return to Emerald Isle with the expectation that Francis would come along. Our life situation had drastically changed, though, and the staff at the Discovery Room advised against upsetting the status quo now that Francis had begun to settle down "after the door episode."

What door episode? Why hadn't I been told about the door episode? Certainly, I should know these things. An aide explained that one day Francis had gone over by the door, laid down on the floor, and declared he would move only if Mary Ann were there. There was no explanation as to why I had not been notified. The bottom line was that travel was not recommended for him at this time.

Helen, Jack, Barnes, and I were in the same duplex that we had occupied in the past. There were new pillows and a new chair. The sun, the sea, the surf, the salty fresh air were the same. No. Same was an impossibility without my Francis.

Helen listened, oh, so patiently, as I related tales of having watched Francis when he threw the tennis ball far into the ocean for Barnes to retrieve, or when Francis dove through a wave and his bald head popped up on the other side, or about how Barnes always stretched his neck and stuck his chin up as he rode the waves like a pro. I saw myself as I had walked to the water's edge to hand Francis a towel and put my arm around his ample, wet waist. Together we laughed as Barnes rolled over and over and squirmed in the sand, which stuck to him like a breadcrumb coating on baked chicken.

It didn't seem right for me to be at Emerald Isle without Francis. Good memories from the past flooded me. I missed him. Afraid of what I might hear, I reluctantly phoned him in the middle of the week.

Ring. Ring. Ring.

"Discovery Room. Hello."

"May I speak to Frank, please?"

"Oh, Mr. Frank is wonderful, having a good day today. I'll go get him," the aide chirped. My heart beat faster, paused, beat, beat, as I waited and waited and waited for Francis to get to the phone. At last, a "hello" from a blank voice, a tentative, remote voice.

I worked to sound cheerful. "Can you tell me what you are doing, Francis?"

"A drum. A topic drum."

"What's that for, Francis?"

Pause. "Odd drum. More effect." Then silence.

Silence.

"I miss you, Francis. I love you, Francis. Are you there, Francis?"

Helen's husband, Jack, got bored with the girl talk and the beach and the limited bar scene, and left after a few days. Creeping fog skittered skyward and Helen and I, packed like mules with chairs, book bags, towels, and sun hats headed to the ocean. The sea.

"I have a saggy butt," Helen announced as we watched cute,

young things with long swishing ponytails and skimpy bikinis parade on the beach. "And have you noticed the vanishing boob act?"

"Whose bosoms, Helen? Mine? Yours? They just point differently that's all. Exercise. Uplifting. Padding. That's the answer," I said.

"Bullshit," she said.

The churned, mushroom colored ocean was calm at low tide. The sanderlings busily dug and picked at whatever they dug and picked at. Little crabs seemed to go in all directions at once as they scurried over the deep tire marks from the trucks that came to clean up the debris from the most recent hurricane. Children were bottoms-up at sizable holes, aimed towards China, until a wave or a call for sandy, soggy peanut butter and jelly sandwiches and lemonade disrupted their projects. Having learned to tune out extraneous noise, I could listen to the slapping surf and the distant buzz of a shrimp trawler interspersed with snippets of memories with Francis at his beloved sea.

Francis phoned and tried to explain a project he was working on. He called it a "squeal" as best I could interpret it. His talk was all gibberish and full of heartbreakingly long pauses. Barnes sensed that I needed comfort and sat by me, his paw on my lap.

It was easy to hang out with Helen. For the rest of the week at Emerald Isle we poked around the towns, tried different restaurants for lunch, soaked up the endless sun. Despite missing Francis, I felt rejuvenated and ready to return home on Sunday.

Hallelujah! Praise the Lord! A message on my answering machine from the Canwell Care Center in Durham informed me that Mr. Frank was next on the list and there would be a Medicaid bed for him within a few weeks. It was not the best facility around, but it was acceptable and nearby. I phoned Carolyn with the good news, the good news that backfired the following day when Canwell Care Center called and said, "We are sorry, yes, sorry, but we don't have that bed for you. Things do change. No, we don't know when we'll have room." The procedure in the world of assisted-living and care facilities, I was reminded, was to give open Medicaid beds to patients already in the facility before considering a new patient, someone like Francis.

When I returned home from my respite at Emerald Isle, I contacted Southern House and a cheerful aide assured me that Mr. Frank was, "Real fine. I think he likes it here."

"Hi, Francis," I said when he got on the phone.

"Hi, hon."

"What'cha doin'?" I asked.

Very seriously, he stammered about some things he wanted "to get going, but not yet." What he described was too vague for me to decipher. It was as if he momentarily lapsed into his previous role as a recruiter in the executive search field, just as he had in the initial interview at Southern House with Pam. I thought that he may not make much sense, but he seemed to enjoy whatever he imagined he was doing. After listening for a bit, I offered up a suggestion: "Let's go to a concert, a foot stompin' event." He laughed, yes, indeed, he laughed as I grinned into the phone.

When I saw Francis next, he was not laughing.

"There. In the corner." An aide pointed to him. There he was. In the corner, with his chin tucked into his neck, his torso collapsed, his legs splayed. I ducked and squinched down like one would do to talk to a little child, or to pat the head of a designer teacup dog, or, if necessary, to rouse a loved one.

"Hi, Francis. Hello. Look, it's me, Mary Ann, and I am here to take you to lunch, okay? We have a lovers' date!"

No response. And then a tiny nod.

It had been over two weeks since I had seen Francis and I was shocked at his deterioration, how thin he was. "He hasn't been eating so good and he's sleeping, sleeping a lot," I was told.

Tea had spilled on his pants. I took him to his room to change. He stood motionless in the middle of his room until I led him over to sit on the bed, tapped his leg and said, "Lift this leg, please." Instead, he toppled over. I hugged his rigid body, felt him tremble.

I switched the lunch venue. Instead of the Steak Saloon, we went to Wendy's where I opted for my comfort food, a plain baked potato. I tried to feed Francis his cheeseburger since he wasn't interested in doing it himself. On the short way back to Southern House, he slept. Fortunately, we had an appointment the following day with Dr. Eveymore.

Of course, silence came in many outfits. We had a new silence. It was blank, dark, dull, not the I-know-what-you-are-thinking communicative silence we shared as lovers, as soul mates. A different silence. Empty, deep, eleventh degree sad.

"You'd better come early to get him ready. He's kind of lazy this morning," the head nurse said when I called to let them know I was on my way to pick up Francis for his doctor's appointment.

"Fine. Let me talk to him, okay?"

"I don't know if he'll come to the phone."

"What? You're kidding me!" I exclaimed.

At last, Francis got to the phone and I told him we were going to Dr. Eveymore today.

"Who that?" Francis mumbled.

I arrived and discovered him collapsed in a chair and alone in the TV room. His pants were wet.

"He pissed his pants four, five times this morning, just kept changing him. Got someone else's pants on but they're too tight to zip. Got him a belt for now," the aide explained.

I woke him up a bit, got his pants changed, found a pair of socks, someone else's shoes, located his glasses at the other end of the hall, and like wobbly drunks, we swayed through the doors that locked behind us, maneuvered past the upscale assisted living dining room, a contrast to the living quarters and dining area of the locked Alzheimer's wing. We passed the library with its vacant game table, entered the fancy lobby, scented by the large bouquet of flowers, and on out to my car.

I made a wrong turn that added fifteen minutes to the drive to Dr. Eveymore's office. Francis didn't care. He nodded off until his head thumped against the window and he jolted awake for a brief grin.

On the examining table, Francis twitched and jerked. His blood pressure was elevated. Dr. Eveymore appeared bewildered. I suggested we get Francis admitted to Durham Regional Hospital for an evaluation. Dr. Eveymore cautioned me that he might not be admitted, a possibility I would not entertain, and told us to wait until he finished his appointments and then he could make the necessary phone calls. We arrived at the hospital and, with a God-given surge of adrenalin, I kept us from falling over as we struggled along the uneven sidewalk from the parking lot to the entrance. I wrapped my arms around Francis, and knew he would have collapsed in a heap if I let go. In no way was I able to describe the relief I felt as I left him in the capable care of the emergency room staff.

A nurse phoned early in the morning and said they had to isolate Francis in the night. He'd hardly slept. He wandered into other patients' rooms. Later in the day, the psychiatrist reported that Francis was Dilantin toxic and should return to baseline after his medications were adjusted. Where was baseline for an Alzheimer's patient riding on a yo-yo? It took seven days for Francis to detox.

"Oh!" said the director at Southern House when I called and informed her Mr. Frank would not be coming back. I could hardly believe my ears when she innocently said, "He was doing very well here." Did she have any real knowledge about his experiences, his episodes, his trips to the emergency room? She continued and asked, "What will you do?"

I chose not to answer. I didn't think she cared.

As soon as I could, I drove to Southern House and asked to look at Francis's medical records. They had been removed from the Discovery Room file. I also learned the staff had phoned Dr. Eveymore days ago and he had suggested an immediate medical appointment and evaluation. I had not been informed of this recommendation, nor had there been an immediate medical appointment.

Francis's duffle bag and personal belongings were gone. The staff could not, would not, tell me anything more than that his things were not there. Gone.

My request that the North Carolina Department of Health Agency conduct an investigation into the care and treatment that Francis had received resulted in a letter of reprimand to the Southern House.

Of course, I would have liked a stiff penalty for the facility and some assurance that such negligence would not reoccur. But all my energy and concern was directed toward Francis's current condition and well-being.

I wandered alone through the Durham Regional hospital corridors for a long time, finding neither a person nor a map to help with directions to my destination. I followed whiffs to the cafeteria and a friendly nurse's aide offered to help me get to Francis's wing. On the door, in big black bold letters, a sign said "Elopement Precautions Area. Please ring bell." After ringing the bell, I was let in. Out of the corner of my eye, I glimpsed the gorgeous silver fringe that I loved to run my fingers through on the back of Francis's head. He sat alone in the activities room, near a clean window with a view of a whitewashed brick wall.

"Hey, you look terrific!" I called out. With a surprisingly steady gait and a small smile, he came towards me, opened his arms so that I could walk right in for a giant hug. He couldn't tell me my name, but he rubbed my back in the old familiar little circles, found my ear and whispered, "I love you."

Always my biggest fear was that he would have forgotten me.

Sammy Smith, the only other patient in the Elopement Precautions wing introduced himself. He was a tall, slender, friendly-looking man of color, and he immediately inquired about my belief in miracles. I paused and then hedged.

"May we pray together, Mr. Frank, you and your lady?" Sammy said.

He took hold of our hands with a firm grip and fervently reassured us that Mr. Frank was on the mend. He urged us go to church and to pray and pray some more to reinforce the miracle. I thanked Sammy for his encouragement and wished him well when he left to allow us to be alone. Then I asked Francis to put his hands over his head to see if he understood what I was requesting. He did it and laughed, a real laugh, a contagious laugh, a beautiful laugh.

This was the first time I had seen my Francis clean-shaven and holding his head up in a long time. It couldn't hurt to offer up a few prayers to reinforce Sammy's conviction that a miracle was on its way. Before I left the hospital, I stopped in at the chapel in the front lobby.

Each day, Francis got better as he detoxed from the Dilantin overdose, stopped being incontinent, lost his twitchiness, and began feeding himself from time to time. He was approaching his baseline.

After Francis had been hospitalized for three days, a Medicare social worker interviewed me and assured me that they would find a bed for Francis, as close to Durham as possible. I realized that the hospitalization that had not seemed remotely possible, had turned out to be the ticket for a bed in a good facility.

"Do you have any choice of facility?" The social worker asked.

"Yes, yes, I do." I was very glad I had done all the footwork looking at facilities.

Barnes came close to my bed and stared at me for a few minutes. As soon as I stirred, he nudged my neck with his cold, damp nose. He knew it was an important day and confirmed his support for me in doggese. It was discharge day from Durham Regional. I frowned and winced as I recalled the wrenching experience from yesterday when, wordlessly, Francis had grasped my arm and tried to go through the hospital door and leave with me. I had wiggled loose and listened for the click and the echo of the locking door that separated us.

Thoughts of the challenges ahead made my gut tighten as I took only shallow breaths. What I had to do was this: find Francis in the locked Elopement Precautions wing, get him discharged from the hospital, drive him to Bridgewood in Raleigh, and get him to willingly go in and get settled into the Alzheimer's wing. During my search for a suitable place I had driven by the Raleigh Bridgewood, but it had looked tired and uninviting and I did not go inside. At least it was located close to home. Unfortunately, there had been no vacancy in the newer Bridgewood facility in Chapel Hill, which had been my first choice.

Francis was ready to leave the hospital when I arrived. As soon as he saw me, he popped out of his chair in the vacant activities room, and came to me, sporting the smile I knew and adored, the customary and jaunty bounce in his step. He appeared slim. The nurse informed me she had been spoon-feeding him most of the past six days. Francis looked so well put together—clean-shaven with a hint of Old Spice, hair combed, pinkish complexion instead of the pale grey I had become accustomed to—that it was doubly difficult to acknowledge he had disabilities. In the car, after he bestowed proper greetings on Barnes, I glanced at the discharge papers. Immediately, I gave them my full attention, as I saw that the fill-in-the-blank regarding his orientation had been altered from "full" to "personal." I phoned the hospital to ask what that meant. It translated to mean that Francis knew who he was but did not understand his surroundings or anything outside his person. Farther down the page I read:

"Prognosis for improvement: none. Chance of improvement: none."

A lifetime of searching for words to describe how I felt at that moment would not suffice.

I altered my plan to stop for lunch, and we drove straight to Bridgewood. What had to be done had to be done as quickly as possible, while I could still cope. The sprawling ranch style façade of the facility was aged red brick, the circular driveway, dark gravel. The place spoke of dingy, drab cheerlessness. I made a feeble attempt to force negative thoughts out a side door and remind myself it was a bed in a secured environment and close to home.

We entered the lobby. "Where's the patient?" boomed across the room as Ramón, the head nurse, greeted us.

Of course, Ramón's greeting pushed me to the edge. Was this a mistake? Did Francis belong with me in the real world and not locked away? Was this for his safety, his best interest? The patient's safety and best interest was the explanation repeatedly used to console caretakers, the soul mates grown weary of watching the downhill race to…where, what end, what finality?

Francis's private, sterile room, with a narrow cot for a bed, a closet, a locker, and a tiny bathroom, was almost at the end of the men's hall, away from the lobby, away from the unoccupied activity room. An old, very tired, but kind looking female aide explained, "We lock everything here, Mr. Frank, otherwise it disappear. We unlock when you want or need something." Four or five dishabille men, one in pajamas, were leaning against the grey hall wall as others ambled over to get a glimpse of the new resident.

We brushed lips as a goodbye. I ignored that Francis reached out to hold me, to keep me, and hastened to the double door entryway. I turned to wave. My Francis was wearing a red and yellow plaid, short sleeve shirt and his white ducks as if we were meeting on a perfect sunny day for lunch in Spring Lake, by his beloved sea, twelve years ago.

In the evening, the social worker at the Raleigh Bridgewood phoned and asked me how to handle Mr. Frank's uncooperative, resistant behavior, and who she could talk to at Southern House for consultation. I was aghast. She reported that Francis refused to get undressed to go to bed, slept in his clothes, and would not get in the shower. What possible advice could I give to a professional social worker? The Mr. Frank she spoke of was a stranger to me, not my Francis.

Later when I called to chat with Francis, I learned that he had tried to run away. "Mr. Frank, he fast," Ramón chuckled. "And, oh, he so strong. Like a fortress. I'm twenty-eight years old, in good shape but, man, Mr. Frank, he so fast, so strong."

"How far did he go, Ramón?"

"Through all the double doors, and 'most to the parking lot. He fast."

A picture sprung into my mind: Francis, wearing his light blue button-down shirt and khaki shorts and his ratty moccasins, his head tucked down, ducking and weaving through the halls, providing a one-man show for the residents who were watching and chuckling, while the head nurse, tall, dark, suave Ramón, dressed in white, loped down the hall, taking giant steps in an effort to capture my Francis.

"He so strong..." Chuckle, chuckle. "Here he come. Mr. Frank, it's your girlfriend, Mary Ann, on the phone. Oh, he smiling now."

In the morning, I checked in with Bridgewood and a female aide told me Francis had been up in the night, with his shirt off, visiting a naked lady in her bed.

"I guessed she thought it was her husband," the nonplussed aide told me.

Of course I worried about the supervision at this residency. More importantly I wanted to know how he could leave his room and wander to the female wing without being detected. The staff reacted as if this were a common occurrence. Even worse was knowing that I didn't have an available alternative care plan for Francis.

Thankfully, a phone call from Bridgewood in Chapel Hill announced a private room available for Francis in Arbor Village, their Alzheimer's unit. I was in Vermont to celebrate my birthday with my family, and Bridgewood would arrange to transfer him. I was glad I had met and chatted with the director when I was doing my initial search. This was wonderful news. The Chapel Hill establishment was upscale, tastefully decorated, cheerful, and most importantly, had an outgoing and friendly staff. The physical layout of Arbor Village, and the attached atrium, was circular. Francis and I spoke on the phone as soon as he was relocated and he sounded pleased with his new surroundings and in good spirits for the first time in weeks. And then he asked me, "When can we go out together, alone?" I assured him I would hurry home from Vermont and be at his side soon.

Of course it hurt—like hell it hurt—when he made comments that suggested being apart was temporary. And it hurt, like hell it hurt, to be powerless about the situation.

During the first couple of weeks after his transfer, the aides asked me to convince him to shower. I remembered that at the Alzheimer's conference it had been stressed that too much emphasis was put on showering. I suggested to the aides that they ease off, and eventually the problem resolved itself. At any rate, Francis seemed presentable to me.

Then a phone call. "You gotta get me outta here, hon. Hon?"

Bridgewood of Chapel Hill resembled a comforting, upscale, vacation hotel, oozing southern hospitality in contrast to the old and tired-looking facility in Raleigh. The gardens in Chapel Hill had been tended to and the shrubs and numerous geranium plants looked healthy. I parked the car and quickly headed towards the entryway to visit my Francis. A chic, young receptionist waved at me. Some patients, sitting in the lobby, hoping something different would happen, responded to my greetings. I was dressed up, as always to meet Francis, and my heels click-clicked on the shiny linoleum as I hurried along the wide, eggshell-white corridor with tall windows overlooking a trellis of roses in a pretty garden. I passed the large, light, clean dining area, took the elevator down to the ground level Arbor Village, and rapped on the locked door. A television was on, the volume very low, and lights were dimmed for group naptime after lunch. In a flash, I found Francis, dozing in a green plastic recliner. The patients all had private rooms, but they were clustered together, hanging out in the large activity room. I patted and jiggled Francis's arm. Numerous sleepy eyes were on us as a giant smile spread across Francis's cheeks and he bounced up to give me a hug.

My impression was that the residents were well treated and cared for here and I thanked God that this environment was available for Francis. Although I had hoped for much more in a miracle, maybe this was the answer to Sammy Smith's prayers.

During his early days in Arbor Village, numerous phone calls came from Francis that resulted in disjointed conversations. As the months passed, our phone conversations diminished in frequency. The phone calls were devastating, knocking me low. They had long pauses and few words, killer phrases like, "You gotta get me outta here, hon. Hon?" that echoed and re-echoed in my head.

After licking his bowl spotless, Barnes would sit by the door to the garage, waiting to get in the car and ride to Bridgewood and have his morning nap in the parking lot. The receptionist would wave or nod in my direction. I would comment about the weather and greet whoever was slumped in his or her wheelchair in the lobby. I would click click click in my heels down the long corridor with its early morning smell of Lysol. I touched the button on the beige wall to open the elevator and be transported to where loved ones were "safe and secure." I rode in the hellishly hot, ninety degree elevator, frequently with a smiley nurse's aide and a terminally ill woman slumped in a wheelchair, her head almost bumping her knees, a small pink bow fastened to her blue-white hair. In the basement, I turned left, away from the wing for the terminally ill and walked down the corridor, trying to avoid looking through the wall of interior windows. But sometimes I looked in at the patients, like people usually stopped and looked in at the newborns in a maternity ward. I would see that Linda quietly stood facing a wall, unable to figure out how to turn herself around. Someone came along and turned her and Linda strolled off to get stuck at a different wall in a different nook in the large all-purpose recreation room. There was Norman, a retired vet, who paced a small circle, as if he were tethered to a short leash. Henry was half toppled out of his wheelchair, a sign that he would leave soon and most likely go to the terminal wing since patients in Arbor Village had to be mobile. Eighty-year-old Ginger sashayed and strutted as she fidgeted with the buttons on her dress, ready to undress and show her imaginary baby.

Where was my Francis?

Half the time I forgot the code to open the door even though I used it everyday. "Hello," I called out, asked for my Francis, smiled as the cheery nurse assured me he was here somewhere, just went by on a walk to somewhere for whatever. When I found him, often he was alone, napping in someone else's room or dozing in a green plastic recliner in front of the television set while a game show host, wearing a gaudy jacket and a spotted bow tie, offered wild and wonderful vacations and prizes to selected winners.

Eighteen months passed. Francis wore baggy sweats and somebody else's ugly shirt. His shoes didn't match. So what? He had been such a dapper dresser, sporting a red or blue silk scarf in his blazer pocket. It was disheartening seeing him unkempt. At long last I understood why it had been so important to my mother to have my Grandma well dressed, her hair combed, and fake jewelry on her wrists and around her neck, during her ten-year stay at the Carleton Nursing Home. Being well dressed presented a façade that helped deny the reality of the situation. It allowed us a chance to believe our loved ones cared about appearances and such things. At home, Francis had been fussy about dressing. As his disease progressed, he re-dressed two or three times a day, wore sweaters over button-down shirts, even in the hot, humid North Carolina summer, until I removed his unseasonal clothes from his sight.

As time passed, I frequently found Francis dozing when I arrived. When I woke him, a slow process of recognition began. His eyes squinched up and then opened wide, wider. His mouth formed a little "O," a precursor to a squishy whistle or just a push of air. On a good day, he puckered up for a smooch. His shaky hands came up from his lap and reached out toward me. I walked into him for a hug. His somber blue eyes pierced me. I wanted to turn away. But I wouldn't.

Dear God, please let me be recognized.

It was impossible for me to stay very long. Some spouses hung out all day it seemed, as they walked, fed, dozed with their loved ones. They sang songs for recreation: "Take Me Out to the Ballgame," "Give My Regards to Broadway," "Itsy, Bitsy Spider." When I explained, with a mountain of feeble excuses about chores and shopping to be done, that I had to leave, Francis put his arm around my waist or held my hand and walked me to the door. Two or three times he grabbed hold of my arm so tightly I knew it would bruise and he tried to maneuver his way out with me. But that was in the early days, fifteen, sixteen months ago. Times gone.

"I love you best, best of all," I mouthed from the other side of the glass door as I cupped my hand to my chin and sent forth a steady stream of in-the-air kisses and Francis waved bye-bye with open, splayed fingers like old timers waved to attract a baby's attention.

One day, Phyllis, a wonderful friend who knew a lot about my experiences with Francis, went with me to visit him. In a polite attempt at conversation, Francis greeted her by asking, "How many miles did you drive?" Then he added, "We're going to take a bath later." And he tossed out some random phrases about the economy.

Driving home Phyllis said, "He looked okay. How do you know what he is talking about?"

"You just know. His cues have become tough for me to decipher. The hardest part is handling his silence, seeing him frown as he struggles to find a way to express himself."

I told Phyllis about George, whom I had met in a bridge group at the senior center. He used to complain because his wife threw mashed potatoes at him. Now, she doesn't talk. I saw him spoon feeding her at Arbor Village and holding apple juice for her to sip. "Rather have the mashed potato deal," he said, as he fluffed the pillows at her back and propped her up again in her wheelchair.

With Francis at Arbor Village, a surge of relief slowly washed over me. I could allow myself short trips to spend time in Vermont more easily, now that I felt Francis was safe.

Of course I tried to believe that Francis was comfortable in his vacantness, but it was impossible for me to ignore thoughts of his mobility decreasing, incontinence increasing, and his diminishing rational mind. Was he scared? Was there any way I could help him deal with his fears?

In Vermont, Barnes and I hiked daily in the park where he concentrated on tracking squirrels and I began to accept the fact that Alzheimer's had captured my Francis and forced him to abandon our life.

Let go and let God

Francis was sitting way across the room facing us when I arrived with Helen, the friend with whom I'd gone to Emerald Isle. I waved, Helen waved, and finally Francis and the lady sitting next to him waved back, but he didn't get up to greet us until I called him. At first he was tentative.

Did he recognize me?

Then he shuffled over, threw his arms around me and whispered in my ear, "I love you so much," as his scratchy beard brushed my cheek.

He reached out to touch Helen's bright blond hair. She and I both felt he couldn't place her but, as always, was being polite. Francis's contribution to the conversation was "ums" and "hums." Without saying anything, he took a packet of photos and a letter from Claudia, his eldest daughter, out of his back pocket and handed them to me. It was too late for Francis to appreciate Claudia's gesture, and I knew he was not able to write back to her. Even before Francis had been diagnosed with Alzheimer's, he sat, pen in hand, bent over blank pages. I had encouraged him to write to his children. By

Christmas time, a year and a half after he moved in with me, he had struggled and ultimately was not able to match up his three children with their respective spouses.

The gist of the letter from Claudia was that she wanted to thank him for the love he had given her as she was growing up. "I have three beautiful children and a wonderful husband, and now I forgive you, Dad, for what you did to our family by leaving us five years ago," she wrote.

Helen and I sat quietly and watched as Francis shuffled, then reshuffled the nine or ten pictures of his three grandchildren. "Cute. Children are cute. Do you know who they are?" he asked.

From the time of our first meeting in 1983, Francis had sought me out, made me feel extraordinarily special. Nine years later, he professed his love and desire to be with me forever. He told me that he had explained it all to his wife and adult children many, many times. "What more can I do? What more is there to do?" he asked as he cried too often at my kitchen table before he left his marital home.

Rationalization had always been easy for me. I figured that Francis did not have a solid concept of time, therefore frequent and short visits from me made more sense than lengthy ones. Three or four words had become the maximum that he uttered during our time together. No longer could I catch any clues of what was on his mind. He patted my back, reached for my hand, kneaded my fingers. He smiled, his adorable, unique smile that crept into his cheeks and forehead. On one occasion, taking baby steps, he followed behind me as I headed to the door to leave. He spoke. Sentences were so rare that it was hard for me to believe what I had heard. It was an unforgettable sentence.

"I'm going to wait. That's w-a-i-t," he spelled it out for me. "I'm going to wait for you here."

Of course, it was hard for me to visit Francis. It was impossible for me not to visit Francis.

At this point I needed to begin to develop a life without Francis as my main focal point. While packing to go to Vermont, my respite zone, I found two pairs of the ugliest socks imaginable—one white pair, one black. Lacy socks with a ruffle at the top. They reminded me of Sunday school days, black patent leather Mary Janes, straw hats with long pastel ribbons, pale blue spring coats. I had bought them at Walmart when Francis was at home when he tried to sort the laundry. Almost everything of mine ended up in his drawers or his closet, except these ugly socks.

Vermont had blue sky, fields of green grass, pastures dotted with cows and horses, little waves on Lake Champlain, Red Rocks Park for outings with Barnes and the dog friends and dog walkers we met there. My grandchildren, who hopscotched across phases of growing up while their parents maneuvered to stay one square ahead, lived in Vermont, and I wanted to be near them. My visits were always short, though. In my head I heard Francis calling and I always drove back to be as close to him as was possible.

His deterioration was swift and impossible to ignore. After a trip to Vermont, I held tightly to his limp hand and helped him get up from the recliner. "We are going on an outing," I announced, "to the parking lot to see Barnes who is waiting in the car." Francis stayed a pace behind me and ignored me. We got on the elevator and Francis stood facing the back wall. Blank. He was blank. I turned him to face forward. I guided Francis along the shiny, white linoleum corridor as we crept toward the double glass doors leading to the outside world. Francis said, "Brrrr," so I knew he had awareness of the change in his environment. It was a glorious sunny day, with a cloudless Carolina blue sky and I wanted to race in a field of tall grasses and scream: "Why? Why us? Why must this be?"

Francis grew more confident in walking and picked up the pace. Barnes was glad to see him and to get out of the car. After a tiny stroll that felt like miles, Francis uttered one word: "Purple." He was acknowledging the color of Barnes's collar. I suggested we go for a ride to, where else, but TCBY. On the way, he slumped in the front seat with his eyes shut tight, like a child who does not want to face the darkness. I kissed his cheek; his lips were sealed. Back in his room, he found my ear and whispered, "I love you."

Turn it over

I was home in North Carolina when the phone rang at seven fifteen in the morning, too early to be a casual call.

"Mr. Frank has hurt himself," Nurse Sandy said.

Francis had been at Arbor Village for a little over a year and recently had shown marked signs of unsteadiness. He was shaky and twitchy. Additionally, I had seen the progression—a regression, really—from full, complex sentences, to simple ones, to phrases, to a single word or two, to a smile, to a bleak blank. Oddly, when Nurse Sandy found him that night, he was sitting in a chair and words flew from him. He explained it hurt so much. He said he loved her. He cried when he moved. An X-ray showed a broken hip. Francis was in an ambulance and on the way to the University of North Carolina Hospital in Chapel Hill when Nurse Sandy phoned me.

I pulled on the first shirt and slacks I could get my hands on, sped to the hospital and raced through the halls, following the arrows to the emergency room, located my Francis, hovered over him as close as I could get without falling on him. He seemed comfortable. His gorgeous, blue eyes smiled when I put my face to his and I knew that he recognized me. He looked like a war casualty, his mouth hanging open, his cheeks slightly sunken under his two-day bristly beard. His bare arm was frail, but he managed to take my hand to his dry lips.

"Kiss me," I said as I bent down farther, and he placed a little pucker on my lips.

"I love you, Francis. Plainly and simply, I love you best of all."

Francis's eyelids fluttered as more morphine kicked in. I sat, stared at the newspaper. Francis laughed and grinned. Once in a while a "who" or "there" or "later" popped out, like a burp. His hand and arm shook as he tried to pull up the flimsy blanket. I guessed he was cold. Cold.

I felt frigid. I wanted to cradle him to my breast, warm his fragile body, carry him away. Flee. Fly.

The lighting was low, everything an eerie pale white. Silence was punctuated by the beeping of a patient's monitor, an occasional phone conversation, the purposeful stride of crepe-soled feet, the slide of a curtain for privacy. The staff in the emergency room was polite, friendly, caring, and oh-so young. They reminded me of children at play, dressed up in their nurse and doctor outfits.

Francis was taken to surgery. I sat and waited for minutes, hours to tick along. An eternity later, it was time to meet the orthopedic surgeon after Francis's operation. The surgery had gone well. The surgeon guessed that Francis had had a nasty fall. Later, I relayed this conversation to the head nurse in the Alzheimer's unit and she huffed and declared that it was impossible, impossible for Francis to have fallen—"We would have heard him." The discrepancy was inconsequential to me; my concern was Francis's recovery.

"We replaced the ball in his left hip socket, a procedure that works better than putting in a pin," the surgeon informed me. "His bone density seemed fairly good." Without stopping for a beat, he added, "The mortality rate in instances like this, with a fractured hip and problems of dementia, is high."

"How high, Doctor?" I nervously interrupted. "What...how high? What do you mean?"

"Twenty percent or higher within a year. It is very important to get Mr. Tomson up and mobile, tomorrow if possible. With a leg brace, of course, so that he will not dislocate his hip."

Francis had such limited, if any ability to understand or follow directions that I could not possibly imagine him getting up and participating in physical therapy.

The doctor continued: "Being in bed makes him a sitting duck for infection, pneumonia, other complications. Just keep telling Mr. Tomson where he is, what has happened, what day it is. Anything. Anything to lessen his confusion."

I stood and stared at the doctor, unable to comment, unable to move.

It had been two years since Carolyn's visit. I phoned her to report that her dad had broken his hip. She already knew, though, because I had asked Bridgewood to notify Francis's three children about any major change in his condition. During the conversation with Carolyn, she told me that Ronald had gone to see his father during the summer while I was in Vermont, and that Francis had not recognized him. How devastating that must have been for Ronald. He had gone bearing gifts—a boom box and tapes that he thought his father would enjoy.

Unfortunately, having been told by the staff at Bridgewood that I was in Vermont, Carolyn misunderstood and thought I had moved permanently and had deserted her dad. I explained my trips to Vermont were only short visits. Carolyn told me she was glad I was with her father.

"You should plan to visit very soon, Carolyn," I told her. I then learned that the three children were planning to visit together within the next three weeks.

"Soon. Come sooner, Carolyn. Will your mom come?" They had

not told their mother about Francis's fall or his surgery.

When I got home, I fell into bed, exhausted, and slept fitfully. I wanted to do everything and do nothing. In my semi-consciousness, I struggled to find something helpful to do, to think.

The next morning, Francis was released from the University of North Carolina hospital and transferred to a bed in the wing for critically ill at Bridgewood.

The head nurse greeted us warmly. I felt nervous and wanted my hand held to enable me to comfort and pass on reassurance to Francis. That was my job, I knew.

After Francis was settled into his bed, a nurse casually informed me, "Mr. Frank has an infected surgical wound. He came that way from the hospital. He will have to stay immobile for a few days."

Her comment set off an alarm in me as I recognized the additional complications that could affect Francis's recovery and level of comfort. Dr. Breakworth, the staff physician, met with me to discuss a comfort-care plan for Francis. He was calm, pleasant looking, middle-aged, and he gave me confidence that he had had plenty of experience in this field. He explained that he would see to it that the procedures for hospice care would be set in motion. I asked for details about hospice and learned that the emphasis would be on keeping Francis pain-free and comfortable. The doctor reinforced the importance of proper nutrition and getting Francis mobile for a successful recovery and added that the mortality rate in instances of fractured hips and dementia was around fifty or sixty percent, not the twenty percent I had been previously told. Mortality. Mortality within a year. Despite Dr. Breakworth's grim news, he had a kindly manner. I felt he would watch out for my Francis.

It was important to get the details. I left Francis in his groggy state in the wing for the critically ill. Click, click, click. I hurried down the long corridor towards the hellishly hot elevator that would take me to the basement, to Arbor Village. Details, I needed details. Questions, questions, questions about Francis's fall bumped into each other in my head.

For once, I remembered the code for the locked door. The head nurse for the night shift stood up at the desk, rewrapped his Big Mac, and came forward to greet me.

"Oh, no, he didn't fall. Couldn't fall. He's a big man. We would have heard him and he's the strongest man here so there was no fight. He's a good man," he said.

The head supervisor promised she would "get to the bottom of this." She said, "You'll hear from me and it will be soon. I'll talk to all the staff. Find out. Call you."

I heard nothing. Not one single word.

After a couple of days, I went to claim his belongings from the Alzheimer's wing. The button-down light blue and white shirts, with their frayed collars, and the meager belongings that had personalized his room—the crossword puzzle books he used to carry, photographs of us grinning with our arms around each other, a photo of his family taken at Claudia's wedding, pictures of Barnes, his huge assortment of pens collected as souvenirs from places we had visited—all of it had been cleared, boxed, and sent to storage.

Francis appeared to be sinking, disappearing. The reports I managed to get about his eating were conflicted. Some nurses said he was eating, one hundred percent. At other times, I was told he was pocketing his food or storing it in his mouth. When I fed him, he opened his mouth, like a bird. Maybe he was chewing or maybe just pushing the food around. I couldn't see him swallow. He looked straight ahead, not at me, not really past me, without blinking, as if he were asleep with his eyes open, as if he were mummified. One time, he fidgeted with his left hand, dropping a pill on his chest. It had been in his mouth. Part of the letter K on it was melted. I brought some chocolates and put a piece in his mouth. He held it there for a long time while my eyes were glued to his Adam's apple.

He swallowed.

"Good," he spoke with a crisp, strong voice. I kissed his forehead and his lips and promised to bring an unending supply of chocolates for him.

My stomach cramped in anticipation of bad news as soon as I saw the blinking light on my answering machine. The message was from Ellen, Dr. Breakworth's assistant, telling me, "Francis had a swollen parotid gland, but since he's been stable for two months we are removing the tubes."

Good Lord. What tubes? What swollen parotid? What was a parotid? What the hell was Ellen was talking about? When I had met with Dr. Breakworth and discussed comfort care for Francis, it was agreed there would be no heroic measures, no life prolonging tubes. It was unspoken, but I understood that the doctor was telling me there was nothing more to be done, no hope of improving Francis's condition. When we had this clinical discussion, I felt oddly detached and at the same time scared but determined to do whatever I could for Francis's comfort.

Ellen answered when I returned her call. "Oh, forget about the tubes. They don't do much good anyway. Patients don't seem to be in much pain when they are shutting down," she breezily declared.

Shutting down. That smacked me. Hard. I felt like screaming at her, "Hey, you, this is a person, my love, my life, my soul mate, my Francis. Not a robot, a wind-up toy losing momentum and about to topple. How dare you, Ellen. How dare you."

And Ellen had continued: "Perhaps Mr. Frank has an abscess or a bad tooth, but I can't get him to open his mouth so I can check. I don't know why, but his compression stocking was too tight. He had some abrasions, which we will treat with light saline solutions. Oh, my, that stocking was on the wrong leg! I'll order an antibiotic to cover all our bases and call you again if necessary."

The phone rang again as I was putting Barnes on his leash so we could drive back to Francis's side. The head nurse and the social worker from the critical care unit called jointly to ask permission to move Frank closer to the nurses' station because he had been trying to get out of bed. He had been bedridden for nine days and was in serious danger of falling.

Francis was sleeping and did not stir when I arrived and dragged a chair up next to his bedside. It was easy to let him be. I wanted to go, go home, go away. Whenever I was home, whenever I was away, I wanted to be back close to him. Wrapped within his arms. Like before. Like way, way, back when.

By law in North Carolina, care conferences are held for patients every six months. Since Francis had been moved out of the Alzheimer's unit and was in the unit for the critically ill, the terminally ill, I was meeting with a new care team. Promptly at 10:00 AM. I arrived.

"Good morning. I am Katrinka, head nurse. You must be Mr. Tomson's daughter. Nice sweater." Katrinka's eyes disappeared when she smiled.

Her comment alarmed me. Francis was sixty-four years old. I was sixty-two and looked every bit of it, probably more. Was head nurse Katrinka on the right case? Confused?

Bitsi, the social worker, welcomed me as she fanned herself, offered me ice water, explained breathlessly that she had been going full tilt all day. She introduced me to the team as the power of attorney. A student was introduced as she came in to observe. I extended my hand; she passed it by.

Katrinka, a very large woman with a porcelain face and red ringlets, started off. "Physical therapy is not happening. It's not working out."

Bitsi said, "Mr. Tomson is not able to follow simple commands."

Katrinka continued, "He can't move himself. The staff is moving his body. It takes three people to move him, big man, from the bed to the Geri chair, to improve his circulation, you know, and to change his environment."

"He wears glasses," Bitsi interjected, looking through her notes, "so we will keep them clean. And arrange for an optometrist if need be. Oh, it is sooooooo hot in here," she said, fanning herself rapidly with her notes. With the exception of Bitsi, everyone in the conference room was wearing a sweater.

"To examine for cataracts, you know," Katrinka added.

I cleared my throat and, in a voice so strong it surprised me, I interrupted: "I have not been able to rouse Mr. Tomson for two days. I think that is the issue to address, not his glasses. How about his meds? I know the Tylenol 3 has been changed to three times a day instead of as needed. How can he let you know when he's in pain and needs medication? Is it too much medicine now? What about the twitching and the jerking? And his Dilantin level? He was Dilantin toxic once before, at Southern House. He had to go to Durham Regional to detox for seven days."

Bitsi got up, mumbled about getting some help and left the room. She returned with Ellen, Dr. Breakworth's assistant, who, yesterday, had left me the message about tubes and an abscessed tooth. I should have told her to stick a piece of chocolate under his nose and he would open his mouth.

Ellen settled into the empty chair on my left and I reminded her that we spoke on the phone yesterday. In a high pitched voice she said, "Ah, well, yes, yes, we are, yes, addressing the issues, his congestion. I will order an X-ray. See about pneumonia."

"Mr. Tomson's Dilantin level, Ellen?"

Ellen sifted through a volume of notes. She could not locate any information about Dilantin.

"He needs glasses to see his food," said Katrinka.

"Is he swallowing or pocketing?" I asked. "He is so frail." The staff was surprised when I told them he had lost twelve pounds in the nine days since his hip operation.

An aide interjected that Frank's operation wound was infected when he came from the hospital.

The nutritionist added, "I will order a menu that is easier for him to manage."

Katrinka grinned broadly, addressed me: "Are you a nurse? You seem so knowledgeable."

Bitsi thanked me for attending.

"Such a pretty sweater," I heard Katrinka say as I closed the door.

At 10:00 PM. the telephone awakened me. It was too late to be a casual call. The night nurse at Bridgewood told me that Dr. Breakworth had asked her to call. Francis's breathing was labored and he was skipping breaths. I raced to Bridgewood, ran down the hall to get to him. He was hot. Very hot. Reaching out. Jerking. Frowning. His gurgling and congestion reminded me of times I have struggled for air with my asthma, and I was afraid he would choke to death on the phlegm that he labored to cough up. I went for the nurse and she suctioned out a large amount of food that was stuck to his teeth and to the inside of his mouth. I bathed his forehead with a warm cloth and stroked the face that I had so often caressed. His once tanned cheeks were pale and sunken. His silver whiskers tickled my clammy hands.

"Everything is all right. I am with you. I love you best, Francis. I love you." That was all I could say. I said it over and over. He heard, didn't he?

I used the phone in the nurse's station to call and give Carolyn an update on her father's condition and I felt compelled to personally call Claudia about Francis's speedy decline. Claudia and I spoke for the first time. Then, distraught, she called me back in a few minutes. "How could it happen so fast?" She was noticeably upset and added that flying made her nervous. Could she drive? she wondered. I offered to meet her at the airport.

Another call from Claudia greeted me when I got home. "Will you ask my father to wait until I can get there, please?"

"Certainly, Claudia."

"My mother said she was sure you would."

As soon as I was back with Francis I told him that his children planned to arrive together to see him in the morning. I relayed Claudia's specific request. No noticeable response came from Francis. Never will I know for sure if he understood any bit of what I explained to him.

At daybreak, Francis was increasingly agitated. His agitation scared me. I asked for help at the nurse's station and was informed hospice personnel could meet with me at two thirty that afternoon and that the intake procedure would take a few days. Good God, what had happened? Dr. Breakworth told me he would arrange for hospice care days ago when we had discussed a comfort care plan.

At the nurse's station I said, "My Francis needs help now, right now. Now." My voice cracked as I tried for control, searched for a Kleenex. A kind hospice volunteer offered to go down the hall with me to Francis's bedside. I sighed with relief. She was totally calm, reassuring, as she explained that his erratic breathing, his twitching, his moaning was common at this stage and that he was probably not aware of it. That he was not aware made me feel much better.

Although it was not his normal day for rounds, Dr. Breakworth arrived at that very moment. He took a brief look at Francis and told me he would order morphine around the clock after he had a chance to examine Francis more fully.

"It will be a day or two at most," he said.

I went home, put a potato in the microwave, got into the bathtub, jumped right out of the bubbles, dressed, rushed back to Francis. As I drove, I ate part of the mealy potato, handed over the rest to an appreciative Barnes.

It was ludicrous to even begin to imagine that Francis could understand anything and yet I found myself talking to him, believing there was a spirit who intervened for us. I perched on a brown metal chair pulled up tight against the bedside. I took deep breaths. Held my breath. His feet and toes felt like ice blocks as I rubbed them to warm them. His forearm was ringed with blue. His face grew pearly. I climbed in beside him, wiggled in as close as possible and lay my head on his chest to listen to the story of our beautiful memories, to be soothed by the melody of his heartbeat. Only my heart thumped.

The empty corridor reeked of hopelessness when I went to find a nurse. Robin, a male nurse who had been so very kind and caring to us for the past few days, sprinted down the hall, his stethoscope bouncing on his chest.

"Is he alive?"

"Barely," replied Robin and he left us to be alone.

I snuggled my head into my love's silent chest and whispered, "I love you, my Francis, best of all."

At approximately 6:50 in the evening, on Thursday, November 9, 2000, Francis died.

Of course I wanted to believe that Francis knew I was with him, that he heard my words and felt my caring. He had begun detaching from the outside world long ago, as the Alzheimer's caught up with him and ruled him. I believe, even in light of his dementia, that he chose to die, as we had lived: alone together.

By the time I went to collect Francis's personal belongings from storage they had been dispersed to Goodwill.

And then a phone call: Claudia wanted to know about the burial. At the time when Francis procured his living will and gave me power of attorney, he had indicated that he preferred cremation. I told Claudia this. There was a pause. I added that they should do what they wanted to do. A long pause. Claudia said, "Is there any money...?" and answered her own question: "I 'spose not."

Francis's family decided to ignore his desire for cremation and to have a burial for him in the cemetery at St. Mary's Church in Clinton, New York—"a little village in upstate New York," as Francis fondly referred to his hometown. For years, he had been telling me he wanted to show me around his beloved Clinton.

I waited, expecting to hear further from the family about the plans. After much deliberation, and not wanting to interfere, I decided to telephone Saint Mary's to see if my Francis had arrived safely.

The funeral director answered the telephone. "Mr. Tomson's family members have all arrived and are here now to discuss the final arrangements."

I sat deadly still. I decided that some day I would travel to Clinton. Alone.

Of course, my Francis,

There is no end.
We go on, plainly and simply,
one decade at a time,
toward forever.
There is no end.

Love,
Mary Ann

And so

My granddaughter was born in June, 2000, a time when it was very difficult for me to be away from Francis.

Four years after Francis died, I went to Rome with a beau. The attraction fizzled.

While on a walk one day with Barnes in Red Rocks Park, I knew it was time to move to Vermont permanently. I telephoned a realtor I had met at a bridge table in North Carolina, asked her to tidy up my house and put it on the market. It sold quickly.

My fourth grandchild greeted the world in November 2006. One more reason for me to live in Vermont.

I stayed at my condo for a year, then I moved into a brand new house only thirteen minutes south of my family.

My granddaughter and I picked up Lulu, a year-old yellow lab, from the Accolade breeder in Pennsylvania, put her in the back of the Subaru with Barnes, and brought her home. At bedtime she curled up to Barnes' backside. Six months later, Barnes died peacefully in the kitchen in July, 2008, after he had relayed to Lulu all necessary instructions about living with me.

Two years later, Lulu and I drove to New Hampshire to adopt Parker, a stray Great Pyrenees. They are best pals. They climb on each other, grunt, race, bare their teeth, and snuggle muzzle. Parker has no interest in learning instructions from Lulu or from me. He is gorgeous. Francis would love him.

*　　*　　*

I am any woman, seventy-four years old. I buy some strawberries on my way to the Hospice Training Program in Colchester. The class is held in the Red Cross building, the same location of the daycare program Francis ran away from a long, long time ago.

Acknowledgments

Many people have had a hand in helping me get this memoir into print. My many workshop leaders gave me courage to keep putting the pieces together.

I would like to thank Claire Samuel for her superb editing.

The Champlain College Publishing Initiative, with intuitive leadership and invaluable guidance by Kim MacQueen, has provided the final backbone of this project. Her team is the cream of the crop. I thank Janina Hartley for her assistance in this production, Martin Simpson for superb design, Nicole Christopher for a topnotch marketing plan, and Jessica Demarest for press releases.

Tobe Zalinger gave me unending encouragement and critical input every step of the way, through the many years I have worked on this book.

Thanks to you all,
Mary Ann

www.ingramcontent.com/pod-product-compliance
Lightning Source LLC
Chambersburg PA
CBHW072135020426
42334CB00018B/1817